Gastric Sleeve Bariatric Diet Cookbook

Delicious Recipes for Healthy Post-Surgery Stomach Recovery and Lasting Weight Loss. Contains Recipes for the 4 Recovery Stages and 60-Day Bariatric Meal Plan

Amanda K. Sanders

© 2024 Amanda K. Sanders. All rights reserved.

No part of this book may be reproduced, distributed, or transmitted in any form or by any means, including photocopying, recording, or other electronic or mechanical methods, without the prior written permission of the publisher, except in the case of brief quotations embodied in critical reviews and certain other noncommercial uses permitted by copyright law.

Table of Contents

Introduction: Embrace the Start of Your New Adventure 1
    Understanding Gastric Sleeve Surgery 1
    Key Nutritional Guidelines Post-Surgery 1
    Setting Achievable Objectives for Success 2

Chapter 1: Introduction to Gastric Sleeve Surgery and Dietary Guidelines 3
    Overview of Gastric Sleeve Surgery 3
    Importance of Post-Surgery Nutrition 3
    Phases of the Post-Surgery Diet 3
    Essential Nutrients and Their Importance 4

Chapter 2: 8-Week Bariatric Meal Plan 6
    2 Weeks Liquid Diet Phase Meal Plan 6
    2 Weeks Pureed Foods Phase Meal Plan 6
    2 Weeks Soft Foods Phase Meal Plan 7
    2 Weeks Solid Foods Phase Meal Plan 8

Chapter 3: Liquid Diet Phase 10
    Creamy Carrot Ginger Soup 11
    Tomato Basil Broth 12
    Silky Butternut Squash Soup 13
    Coconut Curry Lentil Soup 14
    Broccoli Cheddar Soup 15
    Clear Chicken Bone Broth 16
    Velvety Spinach and Potato Soup 17
    Lemon Herb Chicken Soup 18
    Minted Pea Soup 19
    Moroccan Chickpea Soup 20
    Mushroom Barley Broth 21
    Creamy Cauliflower Soup 22

Thai Coconut Lemongrass Soup 23

Sweet Potato Coconut Soup 24

Spicy Black Bean Soup 25

Roasted Red Pepper Soup 26

Tomato Florentine Soup 27

Clear Vegetable Broth 28

Pumpkin Apple Soup 29

Green Pea and Mint Soup 30

Creamy Corn and Poblano Soup 31

Carrot Turmeric Soup 32

Garlic and Herb Broth 33

Miso Soup with Tofu 34

Coconut Carrot Ginger Soup 35

Creamy Asparagus Soup 36

Cucumber Dill Soup 37

Lemon Lentil Soup 38

French Onion Soup 39

Gazpacho 40

Chapter 4: Pureed Foods Phase 41

Mashed Sweet Potatoes 42

Pureed Carrot and Ginger 43

Creamy Cauliflower Mash 44

Pureed Green Beans with Garlic 45

Silky Butternut Squash Puree 46

Pureed Peas and Mint 47

Pureed Lentil and Tomato 48

Smooth Apple and Cinnamon 49

Pureed Chicken and Vegetable 50

Mashed Banana and Avocado 51

Pureed Turkey with Herbs 52

- Pureed Black Beans with Cilantro 53
- Pureed Spinach and Cheese 54
- Pureed Zucchini and Basil 55
- Smooth Mango and Yogurt 56
- Mashed Pumpkin with Spices 57
- Pureed Beets with Orange 58
- Pureed Cauliflower and Cheese 59
- Pureed Lentil and Spinach 60
- Pureed Sweet Potato and Coconut 61
- Mashed Pear and Ginger 62
- Pureed Eggplant and Garlic 63
- Pureed Tomato and Basil 64
- Pureed Squash and Sage 65

Chapter 5: Soft Foods Phase 66
- Soft Scrambled Eggs 67
- Cottage Cheese with Pineapple 68
- Soft Poached Salmon 69
- Greek Yogurt with Honey 70
- Mashed Avocado with Lime 71
- Soft Boiled Eggs 72
- Tuna Salad with Yogurt 73
- Soft Baked Apple with Cinnamon 74
- Soft Tofu with Soy Sauce 75
- Soft Cooked Oatmeal 76
- Mashed Banana with Yogurt 77
- Soft Baked Sweet Potato 78
- Soft Roasted Squash 79
- Cottage Cheese with Tomato 80
- Soft Cooked Lentils 81
- Soft Steamed Broccoli 82

Soft Baked Pear with Nutmeg ... 83
Soft Tofu Scramble ... 84
Soft Baked Fish with Herbs ... 85
Soft Cooked Quinoa ... 86
Soft Steamed Green Beans ... 87
Soft Baked Potato with Cheese ... 88
Soft Roasted Beet Salad ... 89
Soft Mango Smoothie Bowl ... 90
Soft Cooked Polenta ... 91
Soft Steamed Carrots ... 92
Soft Cauliflower Mash ... 93
Soft Black Bean Salad ... 94
Soft Spinach Frittata ... 95

Chapter 6: Solid Foods Phase ... 96

Grilled Chicken Breast ... 97
Baked Salmon with Lemon ... 98
Roasted Turkey Breast ... 99
Stuffed Bell Peppers ... 100
Chicken and Vegetable Stir-Fry ... 101
Baked Cod with Herbs ... 102
Turkey Meatballs ... 103
Quinoa and Veggie Salad ... 104
Grilled Shrimp Skewers ... 105
Baked Tofu with Soy Sauce ... 106
Stuffed Zucchini Boats ... 107
Baked Chicken Parmesan ... 108
Grilled Vegetable Skewers ... 109
Beef and Vegetable Stew ... 110
Chicken Fajita Bowl ... 111
Stuffed Portobello Mushrooms ... 112

Baked Eggplant Parmesan 113
Turkey and Avocado Wrap 114
Chicken Caesar Salad 115
Baked Tilapia with Herbs 116
Veggie and Hummus Wrap 117
Grilled Pork Tenderloin 118
Beef and Broccoli Stir-Fry 119
Baked Chicken Thighs 120
Veggie and Quinoa Bowl 121
Grilled Salmon Salad 122
Baked Falafel with Tzatziki 123
Turkey and Veggie Skillet 124

Chapter 7: Bariatric Meal Preparation Tips 125
Grocery Shopping Tips for Bariatric Patients 125
Time-Saving Meal Prep Techniques 126

Chapter 8: Tackling Common Challenges 127
Managing Food Intolerance 127
Managing Emotional Eating 128
Staying Hydrated and Active 128

Conclusion 130

Recipes Index 131

Introduction: Embrace the Start of Your New Adventure

Gastric sleeve surgery is an effective method of reaching your weight loss objectives, but it is just the starting point. This cookbook, The Easy Gastric Sleeve Bariatric Cookbook, is designed to assist you throughout your recovery journey, offering delicious, nutritious, and easy-to-follow recipes that align with your new lifestyle. Whether you're just starting out or are acquainted with your gastric sleeve, you'll discover valuable insights and practical tips to elevate your experience. Let's embrace this journey together, with a focus on getting to full recovery, one recipe at a time.

Understanding Gastric Sleeve Surgery

Gastric sleeve surgery, also known as sleeve gastrectomy, is a weight loss procedure that entails removing a part of the stomach, resulting in a tube-shaped section resembling the size and shape of a banana. This procedure effectively reduces food intake and suppresses hunger by removing the section of the stomach responsible for producing the hormone ghrelin. It's a transformative surgery that requires a commitment to adopting a fresh approach to eating and living.

The surgery is performed laparoscopically, which means it involves small incisions and the use of a camera to guide the surgeon. This approach typically leads to a reduced hospital stay and quicker recovery time. Nevertheless, it is crucial to remember that gastric sleeve surgery is not an instantaneous fix. It's a tool that, when used alongside a balanced diet and lifestyle adjustments, can help you accomplish and maintain your weight loss objectives.

Key Nutritional Guidelines Post-Surgery

Following gastric sleeve surgery, there will be a significant change in your diet. You must adhere to the nutritional guidelines given by your healthcare team to ensure a successful recovery and achieve long-term weight loss. These are the essential stages and guidelines that you will need to follow:

1. **Liquid Diet Phase:** Immediately after surgery, you will begin with a clear liquid diet to aid in the healing process of your stomach. A whole section of this cookbook is dedicated to recipes for this liquid phase.
2. **Pureed Foods Phase:** After you are able to handle liquids, you will move on to pureed foods. This phase focuses on consuming smooth, easily digestible foods like blended soups and pureed vegetables. There is also an entire section dedicated to exciting recipe options for this pureed diet phase.
3. **Soft Foods Phase:** As your healing progresses, you'll gradually incorporate soft, textured foods into your diet. A dedicated section of this cookbook offers several recipes for this phase.
4. **Solid Foods Phase:** Eventually, you'll slowly incorporate solid foods back into your diet. It's crucial to prioritize high-protein, low-sugar, and low-fat foods. Also, endeavor to chew your food thoroughly and eat slowly to prevent any potential discomfort.

Staying hydrated is essential throughout all phases. Sip water throughout the day, but avoid drinking it 30 minutes before and after meals to maintain a healthy stomach size.

Setting Achievable Objectives for Success

Setting feasible goals is crucial for achieving lasting success. Weight loss following gastric sleeve surgery can be significant, but setting practical and sustainable goals is critical. Here are some helpful tips to help you in setting and achieving your goals:

1. **Set Clear Goals:** Instead of expressing a general desire to lose weight, setting specific goals, such as aiming to shed 10 pounds within the next month, is more effective.
2. **Track Your Progress:** Maintain a journal to monitor your food consumption, physical activity, and weight loss progress. This will ensure that you stay accountable and motivated.
3. **Celebrate Milestones:** Take the time to acknowledge and celebrate your accomplishments, even the ones that may seem insignificant. Reaching a weight loss milestone, fitting into a smaller clothing size, or being able to do an activity you couldn't do before are all significant achievements.
4. **Stay Positive:** Weight loss is a journey that has its share of highs and lows. Remain optimistic and stay motivated despite any obstacles that may arise. Keep in mind that every day presents another opportunity to make better choices for your health.
5. **Seek Support:** Consider joining a support group or connecting with people who have experienced gastric sleeve surgery. Sharing experiences and tips can be very motivating and reassuring.

Ultimately, "The Easy Gastric Sleeve Bariatric Cookbook" is a valuable resource to support you throughout your life-changing experience. By adopting a positive mindset, setting achievable goals, and having access to various mouthwatering recipes, you'll be able to fully embrace your new lifestyle and experience long-term success. Alright, get started!

Chapter 1: Introduction to Gastric Sleeve Surgery and Dietary Guidelines

Overview of Gastric Sleeve Surgery

Gastric sleeve surgery, also known as sleeve gastrectomy, is a transformative procedure aimed at helping you achieve significant weight loss. The surgery removes about 75–80% of your stomach, leaving behind a tube-like structure resembling the size and shape of a banana. This smaller stomach restricts how much you can eat, which helps reduce calorie intake. Plus, it removes the part of the stomach that produces the hunger hormone ghrelin, helping to decrease your appetite.

Typically, this surgery is performed laparoscopically, which involves small incisions on the stomach and a camera to guide the surgeon. This minimally invasive method usually results in shorter hospital stays, less pain, and quicker recovery times compared to traditional open surgery. However, it's important to remember that gastric sleeve surgery is not a quick fix. It demands a lifelong commitment to healthy eating and regular physical activity to achieve and maintain weight-loss success.

Importance of Post-Surgery Nutrition

Good nutrition after gastric sleeve surgery is critical to your recovery and long-term weight loss. Right after surgery, your stomach is healing and can only handle certain types of food. Over time, your diet will gradually progress from liquids to solid foods, each phase carefully designed to support healing and ensure you get the necessary nutrients.

Post-surgery dietary guidelines emphasize high-protein, low-sugar, and low-fat foods. Protein is crucial for maintaining muscle mass and promoting healing. Since your new stomach size limits how much you can eat, every bite needs to count nutritionally. Sticking to your prescribed diet helps prevent complications like nutrient deficiencies, dehydration, and dumping syndrome, which occurs when food moves too quickly from your stomach to your small intestine.

Phases of the Post-Surgery Diet

1. **Liquid Diet Phase**

    - **Duration:** 1-2 weeks

    - **Purpose:** To allow the stomach to heal without the stress of digesting solid foods.

    - **Foods:** Clear broths, water, sugar-free gelatin, protein shakes, and electrolyte drinks.

    - **Tips:** Sip liquids slowly and aim to stay hydrated throughout the day. Avoid carbonated beverages and caffeine.

2. **Pureed Foods Phase**

    - **Duration:** 2-4 weeks

    - **Purpose:** To transition from liquids to more substantial foods while still being gentle on the stomach.

- **Foods:** Blended soups, pureed vegetables, applesauce, Greek yogurt, and protein shakes.
- **Tips:** Ensure pureed foods have a smooth, pudding-like consistency. Continue to focus on protein intake and stay hydrated.

3. **Soft Foods Phase**
   - **Duration:** 4-8 weeks
   - **Purpose:** To introduce more texture into your diet while still being easy to digest.
   - **Foods:** Soft fruits (like bananas), cooked vegetables, scrambled eggs, cottage cheese, and soft meats (like shredded chicken).
   - **Tips:** Chew food thoroughly, eat slowly, and pay attention to your body's signals of fullness to avoid overeating.

4. **Solid Foods Phase**
   - **Duration:** Ongoing
   - **Purpose:** To transition to a long-term healthy eating plan.
   - **Foods:** Lean proteins, vegetables, fruits, whole grains, and healthy fats.
   - **Tips:** Keep prioritizing protein, eat small, frequent meals, and avoid foods high in sugar and fat. Chew thoroughly and eat mindfully.

Essential Nutrients and Their Importance

After surgery, your diet should focus on nutrient-dense foods to ensure you get essential vitamins and minerals in smaller quantities. Here are the key nutrients to prioritize:

1. **Protein**
   - **Importance:** Essential for tissue repair, muscle maintenance, and overall recovery.
   - **Sources:** Lean meats, fish, eggs, dairy, legumes, and protein supplements.

2. **Vitamins and Minerals**
   - **Importance:** Crucial for overall health, energy production, immune function, and preventing deficiencies.
   - **Sources:** Various fruits, vegetables, whole grains, and fortified foods. Your doctor may also recommend specific supplements.

3. **Fiber**
   - **Importance:** Supports digestive health and helps prevent constipation.
   - **Sources:** Vegetables, fruits, legumes, and whole grains (introduced gradually as your diet progresses).

4. **Healthy Fats**

- **Importance:** Necessary for brain health, hormone production, and nutrient absorption.
- **Sources:** Avocados, nuts, seeds, olive oil, and fatty fish.

5. **Hydration**
    - **Importance:** Prevents dehydration, supports digestion, and maintains overall bodily functions.
    - **Sources:** Water, herbal teas, and electrolyte drinks. Avoid sugary drinks and limit caffeine.

In summary, understanding the phases of your post-surgery diet and the importance of key nutrients will help you navigate your new lifestyle successfully.

Chapter 2: 8-Week Bariatric Meal Plan

2 Weeks Liquid Diet Phase Meal Plan

Day	Breakfast	Lunch	Dinner
Monday	Creamy Carrot Ginger Soup	Tomato Basil Broth	Silky Butternut Squash Soup
Tuesday	Coconut Curry Lentil Soup	Broccoli Cheddar Soup	Clear Chicken Bone Broth
Wednesday	Velvety Spinach and Potato Soup	Lemon Herb Chicken Soup	Minted Pea Soup
Thursday	Moroccan Chickpea Soup	Mushroom Barley Broth	Creamy Cauliflower Soup
Friday	Thai Coconut Lemongrass Soup	Sweet Potato Coconut Soup	Spicy Black Bean Soup
Saturday	Roasted Red Pepper Soup	Tomato Florentine Soup	Clear Vegetable Broth
Sunday	Pumpkin Apple Soup	Green Pea and Mint Soup	Creamy Corn and Poblano Soup
Monday	Carrot Turmeric Soup	Garlic and Herb Broth	Miso Soup with Tofu
Tuesday	Coconut Carrot Ginger Soup	Creamy Asparagus Soup	Cucumber Dill Soup
Wednesday	Lemon Lentil Soup	French Onion Soup	Gazpacho
Thursday	Creamy Carrot Ginger Soup	Tomato Basil Broth	Silky Butternut Squash Soup
Friday	Coconut Curry Lentil Soup	Broccoli Cheddar Soup	Clear Chicken Bone Broth
Saturday	Velvety Spinach and Potato Soup	Lemon Herb Chicken Soup	Minted Pea Soup
Sunday	Moroccan Chickpea Soup	Mushroom Barley Broth	Creamy Cauliflower Soup

2 Weeks Pureed Foods Phase Meal Plan

Day	Breakfast	Lunch	Dinner
Monday	Smooth Apple and Cinnamon	Pureed Chicken and Vegetable	Mashed Sweet Potatoes
Tuesday	Mashed Banana and Avocado	Pureed Turkey with Herbs	Pureed Carrot and Ginger

Day	Breakfast	Lunch	Dinner
Wednesday	Smooth Mango and Yogurt	Pureed Lentil and Tomato	Creamy Cauliflower Mash
Thursday	Mashed Pumpkin with Spices	Pureed Black Beans with Cilantro	Pureed Green Beans with Garlic
Friday	Mashed Pear and Ginger	Pureed Spinach and Cheese	Silky Butternut Squash Puree
Saturday	Smooth Apple and Cinnamon	Pureed Zucchini and Basil	Pureed Beets with Orange
Sunday	Mashed Banana and Avocado	Pureed Lentil and Spinach	Pureed Sweet Potato and Coconut
Monday	Smooth Mango and Yogurt	Pureed Cauliflower and Cheese	Pureed Squash and Sage
Tuesday	Mashed Pumpkin with Spices	Pureed Chicken and Vegetable	Mashed Sweet Potatoes
Wednesday	Mashed Pear and Ginger	Pureed Turkey with Herbs	Pureed Carrot and Ginger
Thursday	Smooth Apple and Cinnamon	Pureed Lentil and Tomato	Creamy Cauliflower Mash
Friday	Mashed Banana and Avocado	Pureed Black Beans with Cilantro	Pureed Green Beans with Garlic
Saturday	Smooth Mango and Yogurt	Pureed Spinach and Cheese	Silky Butternut Squash Puree
Sunday	Mashed Pumpkin with Spices	Pureed Zucchini and Basil	Pureed Beets with Orange

2 Weeks Soft Foods Phase Meal Plan

Day	Breakfast	Lunch	Dinner
Monday	Soft Scrambled Eggs	Cottage Cheese with Pineapple	Soft Poached Salmon
Tuesday	Greek Yogurt with Honey	Mashed Avocado with Lime	Soft Boiled Eggs
Wednesday	Soft Cooked Oatmeal	Tuna Salad with Yogurt	Soft Baked Apple with Cinnamon
Thursday	Mashed Banana with Yogurt	Soft Tofu with Soy Sauce	Soft Baked Sweet Potato

Friday	Soft Baked Pear with Nutmeg	Soft Cooked Lentils	Soft Roasted Squash
Saturday	Cottage Cheese with Tomato	Soft Steamed Broccoli	Soft Tofu Scramble
Sunday	Soft Mango Smoothie Bowl	Soft Baked Fish with Herbs	Soft Cooked Quinoa
Monday	Soft Spinach Frittata	Soft Steamed Green Beans	Soft Baked Potato with Cheese
Tuesday	Soft Cooked Polenta	Soft Roasted Beet Salad	Soft Cooked Oatmeal
Wednesday	Soft Scrambled Eggs	Cottage Cheese with Pineapple	Soft Poached Salmon
Thursday	Greek Yogurt with Honey	Mashed Avocado with Lime	Soft Boiled Eggs
Friday	Mashed Banana with Yogurt	Tuna Salad with Yogurt	Soft Baked Apple with Cinnamon
Saturday	Soft Baked Pear with Nutmeg	Soft Cooked Lentils	Soft Roasted Squash
Sunday	Cottage Cheese with Tomato	Soft Steamed Broccoli	Soft Tofu Scramble

2 Weeks Solid Foods Phase Meal Plan

Day	Breakfast	Lunch	Dinner
Monday	Baked Eggplant Parmesan	Chicken Caesar Salad	Grilled Chicken Breast
Tuesday	Turkey and Avocado Wrap	Quinoa and Veggie Salad	Baked Salmon with Lemon
Wednesday	Baked Falafel with Tzatziki	Veggie and Hummus Wrap	Roasted Turkey Breast
Thursday	Grilled Salmon Salad	Chicken and Vegetable Stir-Fry	Stuffed Bell Peppers
Friday	Veggie and Quinoa Bowl	Baked Cod with Herbs	Turkey Meatballs
Saturday	Stuffed Zucchini Boats	Grilled Shrimp Skewers	Baked Chicken Parmesan
Sunday	Turkey and Veggie Skillet	Beef and Vegetable Stew	Grilled Vegetable Skewers

Monday	Baked Eggplant Parmesan	Chicken Fajita Bowl	Stuffed Portobello Mushrooms
Tuesday	Turkey and Avocado Wrap	Quinoa and Veggie Salad	Baked Salmon with Lemon
Wednesday	Baked Falafel with Tzatziki	Veggie and Hummus Wrap	Baked Tilapia with Herbs
Thursday	Grilled Salmon Salad	Chicken and Vegetable Stir-Fry	Grilled Pork Tenderloin
Friday	Veggie and Quinoa Bowl	Baked Cod with Herbs	Beef and Broccoli Stir-Fry
Saturday	Stuffed Zucchini Boats	Grilled Shrimp Skewers	Baked Chicken Thighs
Sunday	Turkey and Veggie Skillet	Beef and Vegetable Stew	Stuffed Bell Peppers

Chapter 3: Liquid Diet Phase

Creamy Carrot Ginger Soup

Prep Time: 15 minutes | **Cook Time:** 25 minutes | **Number of Servings:** 4

Ingredients:

- 500 grams of Carrots (peeled and chopped)
- 1 medium Onion (chopped)
- 2 cloves of Garlic (minced)
- 1 tablespoon of Fresh Ginger (peeled and grated)
- 4 cups of Low-Sodium Vegetable Broth
- 1 cup of Unsweetened Almond Milk
- Salt (to taste)
- Pepper (to taste)
- 1 tablespoon of Olive Oil
- Fresh Parsley (for garnish, optional)

Instructions:

1. In a large pot, heat olive oil over medium heat. Add chopped onions and sauté until they become translucent.
2. Add minced garlic and grated ginger to the pot. Cook for another minute until fragrant.
3. Add chopped carrots to the pot and pour in the low-sodium vegetable broth. Bring the mixture to a boil, then reduce heat and let it simmer for about 20 minutes or until the carrots are tender.
4. Once the carrots are cooked, take out the pot from heat and let it cool slightly.
5. Using an immersion blender or a regular blender, blend the soup until smooth and creamy.
6. Return the blended soup to the pot and stir in unsweetened almond milk. Season with salt and pepper to taste.
7. Place the pot back on the stove over low heat, stirring occasionally until the soup is heated through.
8. Serve the creamy carrot ginger soup hot, garnished with fresh parsley if desired.

Nutritional Information (per serving):

- Total Calories: 120 calories
- Protein: 5 grams
- Carbohydrates: 18 grams
- Total Fat: 3 grams
- Fiber: 5 grams
- Sodium: 200 milligrams

Tomato Basil Broth

Prep Time: 10 minutes | **Cook Time:** 20 minutes | **Number of Servings:** 4

Ingredients:

- 500 grams of Fresh Tomatoes (diced)
- 1 small Onion (chopped)
- 2 cloves of Garlic (minced)
- 1 cup of Fresh Basil Leaves (chopped)
- 4 cups of Low-Sodium Vegetable Broth
- Salt (to taste)
- Pepper (to taste)
- 1 tablespoon of Olive Oil
- Fresh Basil Leaves (for garnish, optional)

Instructions:

1. In a large pot, heat olive oil over medium heat. Add chopped onions and sauté until they become translucent.
2. Add minced garlic to the pot and cook for another minute until fragrant.
3. Add diced fresh tomatoes to the pot along with low-sodium vegetable broth. Bring the mixture to a boil, then reduce heat and let it simmer for about 15 minutes.
4. Stir in chopped fresh basil leaves and continue to simmer for an additional 5 minutes.
5. Take out the pot from heat and let the mixture cool slightly.
6. Using an immersion blender or a regular blender, blend the soup until smooth and broth-like consistency is achieved.
7. Strain the blended mixture through a fine-mesh sieve or cheesecloth to remove any solids, leaving a smooth broth.
8. Season the tomato basil broth with salt and pepper to taste.
9. Serve the broth hot, garnished with fresh basil leaves if desired.

Nutritional Information (per serving):

- Total Calories: 80 calories
- Protein: 3 grams
- Carbohydrates: 12 grams
- Total Fat: 2 grams
- Fiber: 4 grams
- Sodium: 150 milligrams

Silky Butternut Squash Soup

Prep Time: 15 minutes | **Cook Time:** 25 minutes | **Number of Servings:** 4

Ingredients:

- 600 grams of Butternut Squash (peeled, seeded, and cubed)
- 1 small Onion (chopped)
- 2 cloves of Garlic (minced)
- 4 cups of Low-Sodium Vegetable Broth
- 1 cup of Unsweetened Almond Milk
- 1 tablespoon of Olive Oil
- Salt (to taste)
- Pepper (to taste)
- Ground Nutmeg (to taste, optional)
- Fresh Chives (for garnish, optional)

Instructions:

1. In a large pot, heat olive oil over medium heat. Add chopped onions and sauté until they become translucent.
2. Add minced garlic to the pot and cook for another minute until fragrant.
3. Add cubed butternut squash to the pot along with low-sodium vegetable broth. Bring the mixture to a boil, then reduce heat and let it simmer for about 20 minutes or until the squash is tender.
4. Once the squash is cooked, take out the pot from heat and let it cool slightly.
5. Using an immersion blender or a regular blender, blend the soup until smooth and silky.
6. Return the blended soup to the pot and stir in unsweetened almond milk. Season with salt, pepper, and ground nutmeg (if using) to taste.
7. Place the pot back on the stove over low heat, stirring occasionally until the soup is heated through.
8. Serve the silky butternut squash soup hot, garnished with fresh chives if desired.

Nutritional Information (per serving):

- Total Calories: 100 calories
- Protein: 4 grams
- Carbohydrates: 16 grams
- Total Fat: 2 grams
- Fiber: 5 grams
- Sodium: 180 milligrams

Coconut Curry Lentil Soup

Prep Time: 15 minutes | **Cook Time:** 30 minutes | **Number of Servings:** 4

Ingredients:

- 1 cup of Dry Red Lentils
- 1 small Onion (chopped)
- 2 cloves of Garlic (minced)
- 1 tablespoon of Fresh Ginger (peeled and grated)
- 1 can (400 ml) of Light Coconut Milk
- 4 cups of Low-Sodium Vegetable Broth
- 1 tablespoon of Curry Powder
- 1 tablespoon of Olive Oil
- Salt (to taste)
- Pepper (to taste)
- Fresh Cilantro (for garnish, optional)

Instructions:

1. Rinse the dry red lentils thoroughly under cold water and set them aside.
2. In a large pot, heat olive oil over medium heat. Add chopped onions and sauté until they become translucent.
3. Add minced garlic and grated ginger to the pot. Cook for another minute until fragrant.
4. Add the rinsed red lentils to the pot along with low-sodium vegetable broth and curry powder. Bring the mixture to a boil, then reduce heat and let it simmer for about 20 minutes or until the lentils are tender.
5. Once the lentils are cooked, stir in the light coconut milk. Season with salt and pepper to taste.
6. Using an immersion blender or a regular blender, blend the soup until smooth and creamy.
7. Return the blended soup to the pot and adjust the consistency with more vegetable broth if needed. Heat the soup over low heat until warmed through.
8. Serve the coconut curry lentil soup hot, garnished with fresh cilantro if desired.

Nutritional Information (per serving):

- Total Calories: 220 calories
- Protein: 10 grams
- Carbohydrates: 28 grams
- Total Fat: 7 grams
- Fiber: 9 grams
- Sodium: 230 milligrams

Broccoli Cheddar Soup

Prep Time: 15 minutes | **Cook Time:** 25 minutes | **Number of Servings:** 4

Ingredients:

- 500 grams of Broccoli Florets (fresh or frozen)
- 1 small Onion (chopped)
- 2 cloves of Garlic (minced)
- 4 cups of Low-Sodium Vegetable Broth
- 1 cup of Unsweetened Almond Milk
- 1 cup of Shredded Low-Fat Cheddar Cheese
- 1 tablespoon of Olive Oil
- Salt (to taste)
- Pepper (to taste)
- Nutmeg (to taste, optional)
- Fresh Chives (for garnish, optional)

Instructions:

1. In a large pot, heat olive oil over medium heat. Add chopped onions and sauté until they become translucent.
2. Add minced garlic to the pot and cook for another minute until fragrant.
3. Add broccoli florets to the pot along with low-sodium vegetable broth. Bring the mixture to a boil, then reduce heat and let it simmer for about 15 minutes or until the broccoli is tender.
4. Using an immersion blender or a regular blender, blend the soup until smooth and creamy.
5. Return the blended soup to the pot and stir in unsweetened almond milk. Season with salt, pepper, and a pinch of nutmeg (if using) to taste.
6. Add shredded low-fat cheddar cheese to the soup, stirring until the cheese is melted and well incorporated.
7. Heat the soup over low heat until warmed through, stirring occasionally.
8. Serve the broccoli cheddar soup hot, garnished with fresh chives if desired.

Nutritional Information (per serving):

- Total Calories: 180 calories
- Protein: 10 grams
- Carbohydrates: 14 grams
- Total Fat: 8 grams
- Fiber: 5 grams
- Sodium: 220 milligrams

Clear Chicken Bone Broth

Prep Time: 10 minutes | **Cook Time:** 6 hours | **Number of Servings:** 6

Ingredients:

- 1.5 kg of Chicken Bones (raw or roasted)
- 3 liters of Water
- 1 medium Onion (quartered)
- 2 Carrots (peeled and chopped)
- 2 Celery Stalks (chopped)
- 2 cloves of Garlic (smashed)
- 1 tablespoon of Apple Cider Vinegar
- Salt (to taste)
- Pepper (to taste)
- Fresh Parsley (for garnish, optional)

Instructions:

1. Place the chicken bones in a large stockpot and cover with water. Add apple cider vinegar to the water and let it sit for 30 minutes to 1 hour. This helps extract minerals from the bones.
2. Add quartered onion, chopped carrots, celery, smashed garlic cloves, salt, and pepper to the pot.
3. Bring the water to a boil over high heat, then reduce heat to low and let it simmer gently. Skim off any foam that rises to the surface.
4. Simmer the broth uncovered for 4 to 6 hours. The longer it simmers, the richer and more flavorful it will become.
5. After simmering, take out the pot from heat and let it cool slightly.
6. Strain the broth through a fine-mesh sieve or cheesecloth into a clean container. Discard the solids (bones and vegetables).
7. Let the broth cool completely, then refrigerate it. Once chilled, any fat in the broth will solidify on top and can be easily removed if desired.
8. Reheat the clear chicken bone broth as needed. Serve hot, garnished with fresh parsley if desired.

Nutritional Information (per serving):

- Total Calories: 40 calories
- Protein: 8 grams
- Carbohydrates: 2 grams
- Total Fat: 0 grams
- Fiber: 0 grams
- Sodium: 60 milligrams

Velvety Spinach and Potato Soup

Prep Time: 15 minutes | **Cook Time:** 25 minutes | **Number of Servings:** 4

Ingredients:

- 500 grams of Potatoes (peeled and diced)
- 200 grams of Fresh Spinach Leaves
- 1 small Onion (chopped)
- 2 cloves of Garlic (minced)
- 4 cups of Low-Sodium Vegetable Broth
- 1 cup of Unsweetened Almond Milk
- 1 tablespoon of Olive Oil
- Salt (to taste)
- Pepper (to taste)
- Ground Nutmeg (to taste, optional)
- Fresh Parsley (for garnish, optional)

Instructions:

1. In a large pot, heat olive oil over medium heat. Add chopped onions and sauté until they become translucent.
2. Add minced garlic to the pot and cook for another minute until fragrant.
3. Add diced potatoes to the pot along with low-sodium vegetable broth. Bring the mixture to a boil, then reduce heat and let it simmer for about 15 minutes or until the potatoes are tender.
4. Add fresh spinach leaves to the pot and let them wilt in the broth for about 2-3 minutes.
5. Using an immersion blender or a regular blender, blend the soup until smooth and velvety.
6. Return the blended soup to the pot and stir in unsweetened almond milk. Season with salt, pepper, and a pinch of ground nutmeg (if using) to taste.
7. Heat the soup over low heat until warmed through, stirring occasionally.
8. Serve the velvety spinach and potato soup hot, garnished with fresh parsley if desired.

Nutritional Information (per serving):

- Total Calories: 120 calories
- Protein: 6 grams
- Carbohydrates: 18 grams
- Total Fat: 2 grams
- Fiber: 4 grams
- Sodium: 200 milligrams

Lemon Herb Chicken Soup

Prep Time: 15 minutes | **Cook Time:** 30 minutes | **Number of Servings:** 4

Ingredients:

- 500 grams of Chicken Breast (boneless and skinless, diced)
- 1 small Onion (chopped)
- 2 cloves of Garlic (minced)
- 4 cups of Low-Sodium Chicken Broth
- 1 Lemon (juiced and zested)
- 1 tablespoon of Olive Oil
- 1 teaspoon of Dried Thyme
- 1 teaspoon of Dried Rosemary
- Salt (to taste)
- Pepper (to taste)
- Fresh Parsley (for garnish, optional)

Instructions:

1. In a large pot, heat olive oil over medium heat. Add diced chicken breast and cook until lightly browned on all sides. Take out the chicken from the pot and set aside.
2. In the same pot, add chopped onions and sauté until they become translucent.
3. Add minced garlic to the pot and cook for another minute until fragrant.
4. Return the cooked chicken to the pot. Pour in low-sodium chicken broth and bring the mixture to a boil.
5. Reduce heat to low and let the soup simmer for about 15-20 minutes or until the chicken is fully cooked and tender.
6. Add lemon juice and zest to the soup, along with dried thyme and rosemary. Stir adequately to combine.
7. Season the soup with salt and pepper to taste.
8. Take out the soup from heat and let it cool slightly.
9. Using an immersion blender or a regular blender, blend the soup until it reaches a smooth and liquid texture.
10. Return the blended soup to the pot and heat it over low heat until warmed through.
11. Serve the lemon herb chicken soup hot, garnished with fresh parsley if desired.

Nutritional Information (per serving):

- Total Calories: 160 calories
- Protein: 24 grams
- Carbohydrates: 6 grams
- Total Fat: 3 grams
- Fiber: 1 gram
- Sodium: 180 milligrams

Minted Pea Soup

Prep Time: 10 minutes | **Cook Time:** 20 minutes | **Number of Servings:** 4

Ingredients:

- 500 grams of Frozen Peas
- 1 small Onion (chopped)
- 2 cloves of Garlic (minced)
- 4 cups of Low-Sodium Vegetable Broth
- 1 cup of Unsweetened Almond Milk
- 1 tablespoon of Olive Oil
- 1 tablespoon of Fresh Mint Leaves (chopped)
- Salt (to taste)
- Pepper (to taste)
- Lemon Zest (for garnish, optional)

Instructions:

1. In a large pot, heat olive oil over medium heat. Add chopped onions and sauté until they become translucent.
2. Add minced garlic to the pot and cook for another minute until fragrant.
3. Add frozen peas to the pot along with low-sodium vegetable broth. Bring the mixture to a boil, then reduce heat and let it simmer for about 10 minutes or until the peas are tender.
4. Stir in chopped fresh mint leaves and let the soup simmer for an additional 2-3 minutes.
5. Using an immersion blender or a regular blender, blend the soup until smooth and velvety.
6. Return the blended soup to the pot and stir in unsweetened almond milk. Season with salt and pepper to taste.
7. Heat the soup over low heat until warmed through, stirring occasionally.
8. Serve the minted pea soup hot, garnished with lemon zest if desired.

Nutritional Information (per serving):

- Total Calories: 120 calories
- Protein: 6 grams
- Carbohydrates: 16 grams
- Total Fat: 3 grams
- Fiber: 6 grams
- Sodium: 180 milligrams

Moroccan Chickpea Soup

Prep Time: 15 minutes | **Cook Time:** 30 minutes | **Number of Servings:** 4

Ingredients:

- 1 can (400 grams) of Chickpeas (drained and rinsed)
- 1 small Onion (chopped)
- 2 cloves of Garlic (minced)
- 1 Carrot (peeled and diced)
- 1 Celery Stalk (chopped)
- 1 can (400 grams) of Diced Tomatoes (no added salt)
- 4 cups of Low-Sodium Vegetable Broth
- 1 teaspoon of Ground Cumin
- 1 teaspoon of Ground Coriander
- 1 teaspoon of Paprika
- Salt (to taste)
- Pepper (to taste)
- Fresh Cilantro (for garnish, optional)

Instructions:

1. In a large pot, heat olive oil over medium heat. Add chopped onions and sauté until they become translucent.
2. Add minced garlic to the pot and cook for another minute until fragrant.
3. Add diced carrots and chopped celery to the pot. Sauté for about 3-4 minutes until slightly softened.
4. Stir in ground cumin, ground coriander, and paprika. Cook for another minute to toast the spices.
5. Add drained and rinsed chickpeas, diced tomatoes, and low-sodium vegetable broth to the pot. Bring the mixture to a boil, then reduce heat and let it simmer for about 15-20 minutes.
6. Using an immersion blender or a regular blender, blend the soup until smooth and creamy.
7. Return the blended soup to the pot and season with salt and pepper to taste.
8. Heat the soup over low heat until warmed through, stirring occasionally.
9. Serve the Moroccan chickpea soup hot, garnished with fresh cilantro if desired.

Nutritional Information (per serving):

- Total Calories: 180 calories
- Protein: 8 grams
- Carbohydrates: 28 grams
- Total Fat: 3 grams
- Fiber: 6 grams
- Sodium: 220 milligrams

Mushroom Barley Broth

Prep Time: 15 minutes | **Cook Time:** 45 minutes | **Number of Servings:** 4

Ingredients:

- 200 grams of Pearl Barley
- 500 grams of Mushrooms (sliced)
- 1 small Onion (chopped)
- 2 cloves of Garlic (minced)
- 4 cups of Low-Sodium Vegetable Broth
- 1 tablespoon of Olive Oil
- 1 teaspoon of Dried Thyme
- Salt (to taste)
- Pepper (to taste)
- Fresh Parsley (for garnish, optional)

Instructions:

1. In a large pot, heat olive oil over medium heat. Add chopped onions and sauté until they become translucent.
2. Add minced garlic to the pot and cook for another minute until fragrant.
3. Add sliced mushrooms to the pot and cook until they release their moisture and start to brown, about 5-7 minutes.
4. Stir in pearl barley and dried thyme. Cook for another minute to toast the barley.
5. Pour in low-sodium vegetable broth and bring the mixture to a boil. Reduce heat to low, cover the pot, and let it simmer for about 30-35 minutes or until the barley is tender.
6. Season the broth with salt and pepper to taste.
7. Using an immersion blender or a regular blender, blend the soup partially to achieve a chunky texture.
8. Heat the soup over low heat until warmed through.
9. Serve the mushroom barley broth hot, garnished with fresh parsley if desired.

Nutritional Information (per serving):

- Total Calories: 190 calories
- Protein: 8 grams
- Carbohydrates: 32 grams
- Total Fat: 3 grams
- Fiber: 6 grams
- Sodium: 180 milligrams

Creamy Cauliflower Soup

Prep Time: 10 minutes | **Cook Time:** 25 minutes | **Number of Servings:** 4

Ingredients:

- 1 medium Cauliflower Head (cut into florets)
- 1 small Onion (chopped)
- 2 cloves of Garlic (minced)
- 4 cups of Low-Sodium Vegetable Broth
- 1 cup of Unsweetened Almond Milk
- 1 tablespoon of Olive Oil
- Salt (to taste)
- Pepper (to taste)
- Fresh Chives (for garnish, optional)

Instructions:

1. In a large pot, heat olive oil over medium heat. Add chopped onions and sauté until they become translucent.
2. Add minced garlic to the pot and cook for another minute until fragrant.
3. Add cauliflower florets to the pot along with low-sodium vegetable broth. Bring the mixture to a boil, then reduce heat and let it simmer for about 15-20 minutes or until the cauliflower is tender.
4. Using an immersion blender or a regular blender, blend the soup until smooth and creamy.
5. Return the blended soup to the pot and stir in unsweetened almond milk. Season with salt and pepper to taste.
6. Heat the soup over low heat until warmed through, stirring occasionally.
7. Serve the creamy cauliflower soup hot, garnished with fresh chives if desired.

Nutritional Information (per serving):

- Total Calories: 120 calories
- Protein: 6 grams
- Carbohydrates: 14 grams
- Total Fat: 4 grams
- Fiber: 5 grams
- Sodium: 180 milligrams

Thai Coconut Lemongrass Soup

Prep Time: 15 minutes | **Cook Time:** 25 minutes | **Number of Servings:** 4

Ingredients:

- 1 can (400 ml) of Coconut Milk
- 4 cups of Low-Sodium Vegetable Broth
- 200 grams of Firm Tofu (cubed)
- 1 stalk of Lemongrass (sliced)
- 2 cloves of Garlic (minced)
- 1 small Red Chili (sliced, optional for heat)
- 1 inch piece of Fresh Ginger (sliced)
- 1 Carrot (julienned)
- 1 Red Bell Pepper (sliced)
- 1 tablespoon of Soy Sauce (low-sodium)
- 1 tablespoon of Olive Oil
- Salt (to taste)
- Pepper (to taste)
- Fresh Cilantro (for garnish, optional)
- Lime wedges (for serving, optional)

Instructions:

1. In a large pot, heat olive oil over medium heat. Add minced garlic, sliced lemongrass, sliced ginger, and sliced red chili (if using). Sauté for 1-2 minutes until fragrant.
2. Pour in low-sodium vegetable broth and bring it to a simmer.
3. Add cubed tofu, julienned carrot, and sliced red bell pepper to the pot. Cook for about 5-7 minutes until the vegetables are tender.
4. Stir in coconut milk and low-sodium soy sauce. Season with salt and pepper to taste.
5. Simmer the soup for an additional 5 minutes to blend the flavors.
6. Take out the lemongrass stalk and ginger slices from the soup before serving.
7. Ladle the Thai coconut lemongrass soup into bowls. Garnish with fresh cilantro and serve with lime wedges on the side.

Nutritional Information (per serving):

- Total Calories: 180 calories
- Protein: 10 grams
- Carbohydrates: 10 grams
- Total Fat: 12 grams
- Fiber: 3 grams
- Sodium: 160 milligrams

Sweet Potato Coconut Soup

Prep Time: 15 minutes | **Cook Time:** 30 minutes | **Number of Servings:** 4

Ingredients:

- 2 medium Sweet Potatoes (peeled and diced)
- 1 can (400 ml) of Coconut Milk (unsweetened)
- 4 cups of Low-Sodium Vegetable Broth
- 1 small Onion (chopped)
- 2 cloves of Garlic (minced)
- 1 tablespoon of Olive Oil
- 1 teaspoon of Ground Cumin
- 1 teaspoon of Ground Turmeric
- Salt (to taste)
- Pepper (to taste)
- Fresh Cilantro (for garnish, optional)

Instructions:

1. In a large pot, heat olive oil over medium heat. Add chopped onions and sauté until they become translucent.
2. Add minced garlic to the pot and cook for another minute until fragrant.
3. Add diced sweet potatoes to the pot along with ground cumin and ground turmeric. Sauté for 2-3 minutes to coat the sweet potatoes with the spices.
4. Pour in low-sodium vegetable broth and bring the mixture to a boil. Reduce heat to low, cover the pot, and let it simmer for about 20-25 minutes or until the sweet potatoes are tender.
5. Using an immersion blender or a regular blender, blend the soup until smooth and creamy.
6. Return the blended soup to the pot and stir in coconut milk. Season with salt and pepper to taste.
7. Heat the soup over low heat until warmed through, stirring occasionally.
8. Serve the sweet potato coconut soup hot, garnished with fresh cilantro if desired.

Nutritional Information (per serving):

- Total Calories: 220 calories
- Protein: 4 grams
- Carbohydrates: 20 grams
- Total Fat: 15 grams
- Fiber: 4 grams
- Sodium: 200 milligrams

Spicy Black Bean Soup

Prep Time: 15 minutes | **Cook Time:** 30 minutes | **Number of Servings:** 4

Ingredients:

- 2 cans (400 grams each) of Black Beans (rinsed and drained)
- 4 cups of Low-Sodium Vegetable Broth
- 1 Onion (chopped)
- 2 cloves of Garlic (minced)
- 1 Red Bell Pepper (diced)
- 1 Jalapeño Pepper (seeded and minced)
- 1 teaspoon of Ground Cumin
- 1 teaspoon of Chili Powder
- 1/2 teaspoon of Smoked Paprika
- 1 tablespoon of Olive Oil
- Salt (to taste)
- Pepper (to taste)
- Fresh Cilantro (for garnish, optional)
- Lime wedges (for serving, optional)

Instructions:

1. In a large pot, heat olive oil over medium heat. Add chopped onions, minced garlic, diced red bell pepper, and minced jalapeño pepper. Sauté until the vegetables are softened, about 5-7 minutes.
2. Add ground cumin, chili powder, and smoked paprika to the pot. Stir adequately to coat the vegetables with the spices.
3. Pour in low-sodium vegetable broth and bring the mixture to a boil.
4. Reduce heat to low and add the rinsed and drained black beans to the pot. Simmer for about 15-20 minutes to allow the flavors to meld together.
5. Using an immersion blender or a regular blender, blend a portion of the soup until smooth while leaving some beans and vegetables chunky for texture.
6. Season the soup with salt and pepper to taste.
7. Heat the soup over low heat until warmed through.
8. Serve the spicy black bean soup hot, garnished with fresh cilantro and lime wedges if desired.

Nutritional Information (per serving):

- Total Calories: 180 calories
- Protein: 9 grams
- Carbohydrates: 28 grams
- Total Fat: 3 grams
- Fiber: 10 grams
- Sodium: 220 milligrams

Roasted Red Pepper Soup

Prep Time: 15 minutes | **Cook Time:** 30 minutes | **Number of Servings:** 4

Ingredients:

- 4 Red Bell Peppers (roasted and peeled)
- 1 Onion (chopped)
- 2 cloves Garlic (minced)
- 4 cups Low-Sodium Vegetable Broth
- 1 tablespoon Olive Oil
- 1 teaspoon Smoked Paprika
- 1 teaspoon Ground Cumin
- 1 Carrot (peeled and diced)
- 1 Celery Stalk (diced)
- Salt (to taste)
- Pepper (to taste)
- Fresh Basil (for garnish, optional)

Instructions:

1. Preheat the oven to 400 degrees Fahrenheit. Place the red bell peppers on a baking sheet and roast for 20 minutes, or until the skins are blackened. Transfer the roasted peppers to a bowl, cover, and let them steam for 10 minutes. Peel the skins and take out the seeds.
2. In a large pot, heat olive oil over medium heat. Add chopped onions, minced garlic, diced carrot, and diced celery. Sauté until the vegetables are softened, about 5-7 minutes.
3. Add the smoked paprika and ground cumin to the pot. Stir adequately to coat the vegetables with the spices.
4. Add the peeled and roasted red bell peppers to the pot. Pour in the low-sodium vegetable broth and bring the mixture to a boil.
5. Reduce the heat and let the soup simmer for 10-15 minutes.
6. Using an immersion blender or a regular blender, blend the soup until it reaches a smooth, liquid consistency.
7. Season the soup with salt and pepper to taste.
8. Heat the soup over low heat until warmed through.
9. Serve the roasted red pepper soup hot, garnished with fresh basil if desired.

Nutritional Information (per serving):

- Total Calories: 120 calories
- Protein: 3 grams
- Carbohydrates: 20 grams
- Total Fat: 3 grams
- Fiber: 4 grams
- Sodium: 180 milligrams

Tomato Florentine Soup

Prep Time: 10 minutes | **Cook Time:** 20 minutes | **Servings:** 4

Ingredients

- 1 tablespoon olive oil
- 1 medium onion, diced
- 2 cloves garlic, minced
- 4 cups low-sodium vegetable broth
- 2 cups fresh tomatoes, chopped
- 1 cup baby spinach, chopped
- 1 cup cooked white beans (low-sodium, rinsed and drained)
- 1 teaspoon dried basil
- 1 teaspoon dried oregano
- 1 teaspoon dried thyme
- 1/4 teaspoon black pepper

Instructions

1. Heat the olive oil in a large pot over medium heat.
2. Add the diced onion and cook until soft, about 5 minutes.
3. Add the minced garlic and cook for another minute.
4. Stir in the chopped tomatoes, dried basil, dried oregano, dried thyme, and black pepper. Cook for 5 minutes, allowing the tomatoes to break down slightly.
5. Pour in the low-sodium vegetable broth and bring the mixture to a boil.
6. Add the cooked white beans and chopped baby spinach. Simmer for 10 minutes.
7. Use an immersion blender to puree the soup until smooth, ensuring a liquid consistency suitable for the liquid diet phase.
8. Serve warm.

Nutritional Information (per serving)

- **Total Calories:** 150 kcal
- **Protein:** 6 g
- **Carbohydrates:** 20 g
- **Total Fat:** 3 g
- **Fiber:** 6 g
- **Sodium:** 150 mg

Clear Vegetable Broth

Prep Time: 10 minutes | **Cook Time:** 45 minutes | **Servings:** 4

Ingredients

- 1 tablespoon olive oil
- 1 medium onion, diced
- 2 cloves garlic, minced
- 2 medium carrots, sliced
- 2 celery stalks, sliced
- 1 small zucchini, diced
- 1 cup baby spinach, chopped
- 6 cups water
- 1 teaspoon dried thyme
- 1 teaspoon dried parsley
- 1/4 teaspoon black pepper
- 1 bay leaf

Instructions

1. Heat the olive oil in a large pot over medium heat.
2. Add the diced onion and cook until soft, about 5 minutes.
3. Add the minced garlic and cook for another minute.
4. Add the sliced carrots, sliced celery, and diced zucchini. Cook for 5 minutes, stirring occasionally.
5. Pour in the water and add the dried thyme, dried parsley, black pepper, and bay leaf. Bring to a boil.
6. Reduce heat and simmer for 30 minutes.
7. Add the chopped baby spinach and simmer for an additional 5 minutes.
8. Strain the broth through a fine-mesh sieve or cheesecloth to ensure a clear liquid consistency suitable for the liquid diet phase.
9. Serve warm.

Nutritional Information (per serving)

- **Total Calories:** 50 kcal
- **Protein:** 2 g
- **Carbohydrates:** 10 g
- **Total Fat:** 1 g
- **Fiber:** 2 g
- **Sodium:** 50 mg

Pumpkin Apple Soup

Prep Time: 10 minutes | **Cook Time:** 30 minutes | **Servings:** 4

Ingredients

- 1 tablespoon olive oil
- 1 medium onion, diced
- 2 cloves garlic, minced
- 2 cups pumpkin puree (unsweetened)
- 1 large apple, peeled, cored, and diced
- 4 cups low-sodium vegetable broth
- 1 teaspoon ground cinnamon
- 1/2 teaspoon ground nutmeg
- 1/4 teaspoon black pepper
- 1/2 cup plain Greek yogurt (optional, for added protein)

Instructions

1. Heat the olive oil in a large pot over medium heat.
2. Add the diced onion and cook until soft, about 5 minutes.
3. Add the minced garlic and cook for another minute.
4. Stir in the pumpkin puree, diced apple, ground cinnamon, ground nutmeg, and black pepper.
5. Pour in the low-sodium vegetable broth and bring the mixture to a boil.
6. Reduce the heat and simmer for 20 minutes, until the apple is tender.
7. Use an immersion blender to puree the soup until smooth, ensuring a liquid consistency suitable for the liquid diet phase.
8. If using, stir in the plain Greek yogurt for added protein and blend again until smooth.
9. Serve warm.

Nutritional Information (per serving)

- **Total Calories:** 90 kcal
- **Protein:** 4 g
- **Carbohydrates:** 18 g
- **Total Fat:** 2 g
- **Fiber:** 4 g
- **Sodium:** 100 mg

Green Pea and Mint Soup

Prep Time: 10 minutes | **Cook Time:** 20 minutes | **Servings:** 4

Ingredients

- 1 tablespoon olive oil
- 1 medium onion, diced
- 2 cloves garlic, minced
- 4 cups low-sodium vegetable broth
- 4 cups fresh or frozen green peas
- 1/4 cup fresh mint leaves, chopped
- 1/4 teaspoon black pepper
- 1/2 cup plain Greek yogurt (optional, for added protein)

Instructions

1. Heat the olive oil in a large pot over medium heat.
2. Add the diced onion and cook until soft, about 5 minutes.
3. Add the minced garlic and cook for another minute.
4. Pour in the low-sodium vegetable broth and bring to a boil.
5. Add the green peas and chopped fresh mint leaves. Simmer for 10 minutes.
6. Add the black pepper and use an immersion blender to puree the soup until smooth, ensuring a liquid consistency suitable for the liquid diet phase.
7. If using, stir in the plain Greek yogurt for added protein and blend again until smooth.
8. Serve warm.

Nutritional Information (per serving)

- **Total Calories:** 110 kcal
- **Protein:** 7 g
- **Carbohydrates:** 18 g
- **Total Fat:** 2 g
- **Fiber:** 6 g
- **Sodium:** 80 mg

Creamy Corn and Poblano Soup

Prep Time: 10 minutes | **Cook Time:** 25 minutes | **Servings:** 4

Ingredients

- 1 tablespoon olive oil
- 1 medium onion, diced
- 2 cloves garlic, minced
- 2 poblano peppers, roasted, peeled, and diced
- 4 cups low-sodium vegetable broth
- 3 cups corn kernels (fresh or frozen)
- 1 teaspoon ground cumin
- 1/4 teaspoon black pepper
- 1/2 cup plain Greek yogurt (optional, for added protein)

Instructions

1. Heat the olive oil in a large pot over medium heat.
2. Add the diced onion and cook until soft, about 5 minutes.
3. Add the minced garlic and cook for another minute.
4. Stir in the diced roasted poblano peppers, corn kernels, ground cumin, and black pepper.
5. Pour in the low-sodium vegetable broth and bring the mixture to a boil.
6. Reduce the heat and simmer for 15 minutes, until the corn is tender.
7. Use an immersion blender to puree the soup until smooth, ensuring a liquid consistency suitable for the liquid diet phase.
8. If using, stir in the plain Greek yogurt for added protein and blend again until smooth.
9. Serve warm.

Nutritional Information (per serving)

- **Total Calories:** 120 kcal
- **Protein:** 6 g
- **Carbohydrates:** 22 g
- **Total Fat:** 2 g
- **Fiber:** 4 g
- **Sodium:** 90 mg

Carrot Turmeric Soup

Prep Time: 10 minutes | **Cook Time:** 25 minutes | **Servings:** 4

Ingredients

- 1 tablespoon olive oil
- 1 medium onion, diced
- 2 cloves garlic, minced
- 1 teaspoon ground turmeric
- 1/2 teaspoon ground cumin
- 6 large carrots, peeled and sliced
- 4 cups low-sodium vegetable broth
- 1/4 teaspoon black pepper
- 1/2 cup plain Greek yogurt (optional, for added protein)

Instructions

1. Heat the olive oil in a large pot over medium heat.
2. Add the diced onion and cook until soft, about 5 minutes.
3. Add the minced garlic and cook for another minute.
4. Stir in the ground turmeric and ground cumin, cooking for 1 minute to release their flavors.
5. Add the sliced carrots and pour in the low-sodium vegetable broth. Bring the mixture to a boil.
6. Reduce the heat and simmer for 20 minutes, until the carrots are tender.
7. Add the black pepper and use an immersion blender to puree the soup until smooth, ensuring a liquid consistency suitable for the liquid diet phase.
8. If using, stir in the plain Greek yogurt for added protein and blend again until smooth.
9. Serve warm.

Nutritional Information (per serving)

- **Total Calories:** 100 kcal
- **Protein:** 4 g
- **Carbohydrates:** 18 g
- **Total Fat:** 2 g
- **Fiber:** 4 g
- **Sodium:** 80 mg

Garlic and Herb Broth

Prep Time: 10 minutes | **Cook Time:** 30 minutes | **Servings:** 4

Ingredients

- 1 tablespoon olive oil
- 1 medium onion, diced
- 6 cloves garlic, minced
- 1 teaspoon dried thyme
- 1 teaspoon dried rosemary
- 1 teaspoon dried parsley
- 1 bay leaf
- 6 cups water
- 1/4 teaspoon black pepper

Instructions

1. Heat the olive oil in a large pot over medium heat.
2. Add the diced onion and cook until soft, about 5 minutes.
3. Add the minced garlic and cook for another minute.
4. Stir in the dried thyme, dried rosemary, dried parsley, and black pepper.
5. Pour in the water and add the bay leaf. Bring the mixture to a boil.
6. Reduce the heat and simmer for 25 minutes.
7. Strain the broth through a fine-mesh sieve or cheesecloth to ensure a clear liquid consistency suitable for the liquid diet phase.
8. Serve warm.

Nutritional Information (per serving)

- **Total Calories:** 30 kcal
- **Protein:** 1 g
- **Carbohydrates:** 5 g
- **Total Fat:** 1 g
- **Fiber:** 1 g
- **Sodium:** 15 mg

Miso Soup with Tofu

Prep Time: 10 minutes | **Cook Time:** 15 minutes | **Servings:** 4

Ingredients

- 6 cups water
- 1/4 cup white miso paste
- 1 cup silken tofu, diced
- 1/2 cup green onions, sliced
- 1 tablespoon dried wakame seaweed
- 1 teaspoon sesame oil (optional, for healthy fats)

Instructions

1. In a large pot, bring the water to a gentle simmer over medium heat.
2. Place the white miso paste in a small bowl and add a ladle of the warm water from the pot. Stir until the miso paste is completely dissolved, then return the mixture to the pot.
3. Add the diced silken tofu and dried wakame seaweed to the pot. Simmer for 5 minutes, until the seaweed rehydrates and the tofu is heated through.
4. Stir in the sliced green onions and simmer for an additional 2 minutes.
5. If using, add the sesame oil for healthy fats, stirring to combine.
6. Use an immersion blender to puree the soup until smooth, ensuring a liquid consistency suitable for the liquid diet phase.
7. Serve warm.

Nutritional Information (per serving)

- **Total Calories:** 60 kcal
- **Protein:** 5 g
- **Carbohydrates:** 6 g
- **Total Fat:** 2 g
- **Fiber:** 1 g
- **Sodium:** 150 mg

Coconut Carrot Ginger Soup

Prep Time: 10 minutes | **Cook Time:** 25 minutes | **Servings:** 4

Ingredients

- 1 tablespoon coconut oil
- 1 medium onion, diced
- 2 cloves garlic, minced
- 1 tablespoon fresh ginger, grated
- 6 large carrots, peeled and sliced
- 4 cups low-sodium vegetable broth
- 1 cup light coconut milk
- 1/4 teaspoon black pepper
- 1/2 teaspoon ground turmeric

Instructions

1. Heat the coconut oil in a large pot over medium heat.
2. Add the diced onion and cook until soft, about 5 minutes.
3. Add the minced garlic and grated fresh ginger, cooking for another minute.
4. Stir in the sliced carrots, ground turmeric, and black pepper.
5. Pour in the low-sodium vegetable broth and bring the mixture to a boil.
6. Reduce the heat and simmer for 20 minutes, until the carrots are tender.
7. Stir in the light coconut milk.
8. Use an immersion blender to puree the soup until smooth, ensuring a liquid consistency suitable for the liquid diet phase.
9. Serve warm.

Nutritional Information (per serving)

- **Total Calories:** 120 kcal
- **Protein:** 2 g
- **Carbohydrates:** 15 g
- **Total Fat:** 6 g
- **Fiber:** 4 g
- **Sodium:** 70 mg

Creamy Asparagus Soup

Prep Time: 10 minutes | **Cook Time:** 20 minutes | **Servings:** 4

Ingredients

- 1 tablespoon olive oil
- 1 medium onion, diced
- 2 cloves garlic, minced
- 1 pound asparagus, trimmed and cut into 1-inch pieces
- 4 cups low-sodium vegetable broth
- 1/2 cup plain Greek yogurt (optional, for added protein)
- 1/4 teaspoon black pepper
- 1/2 teaspoon dried thyme

Instructions

1. Heat the olive oil in a large pot over medium heat.
2. Add the diced onion and cook until soft, about 5 minutes.
3. Add the minced garlic and cook for another minute.
4. Stir in the asparagus pieces and dried thyme, cooking for an additional 5 minutes.
5. Pour in the low-sodium vegetable broth and bring the mixture to a boil.
6. Reduce the heat and simmer for 10 minutes, until the asparagus is tender.
7. Use an immersion blender to puree the soup until smooth, ensuring a liquid consistency suitable for the liquid diet phase.
8. If using, stir in the plain Greek yogurt for added protein and blend again until smooth.
9. Add the black pepper and adjust seasoning as needed.
10. Serve warm.

Nutritional Information (per serving)

- **Total Calories:** 90 kcal
- **Protein:** 6 g
- **Carbohydrates:** 10 g
- **Total Fat:** 3 g
- **Fiber:** 3 g
- **Sodium:** 70 mg

Cucumber Dill Soup

Prep Time: 10 minutes | **Cook Time:** 0 minutes | **Servings:** 4

Ingredients

- 2 large cucumbers, peeled and chopped
- 1 cup plain Greek yogurt
- 1/4 cup fresh dill, chopped
- 1 tablespoon lemon juice
- 1/4 teaspoon ground black pepper
- 1/2 cup water (adjust for desired consistency)
- Salt to taste

Instructions

1. In a blender or food processor, put together the chopped cucumbers, plain Greek yogurt, fresh dill, lemon juice, ground black pepper, and water.
2. Blend until smooth, adding more water if necessary to achieve a liquid consistency suitable for the liquid diet phase.
3. Season with salt to taste.
4. If the soup is too thick, add more water and blend again until desired consistency is reached.
5. Chill the soup in the refrigerator for at least 1 hour before serving.
6. Serve cold garnished with additional dill if desired.

Nutritional Information (per serving)

- **Total Calories:** 60 kcal
- **Protein:** 6 g
- **Carbohydrates:** 8 g
- **Total Fat:** 1 g
- **Fiber:** 1 g
- **Sodium:** 30 mg

Lemon Lentil Soup

Prep Time: 10 minutes | **Cook Time:** 30 minutes | **Servings:** 4

Ingredients

- 1 cup dried brown lentils, rinsed
- 6 cups low-sodium vegetable broth
- 1 medium onion, finely chopped
- 2 cloves garlic, minced
- 1 teaspoon ground cumin
- 1/2 teaspoon ground turmeric
- 1/4 teaspoon ground black pepper
- Zest of 1 lemon
- Juice of 1 lemon
- 2 tablespoons chopped fresh parsley
- Salt to taste

Instructions

1. In a large pot, put together the rinsed brown lentils and low-sodium vegetable broth. Bring to a boil over medium-high heat.
2. Reduce the heat to low, cover, and simmer for 20-25 minutes, or until the lentils are tender.
3. In a separate pan, heat a bit of water or broth over medium heat. Add the finely chopped onion and cook until softened, about 5-7 minutes.
4. Add the minced garlic, ground cumin, ground turmeric, and ground black pepper to the onions. Cook for an additional 1-2 minutes until fragrant.
5. Transfer the onion and spice mixture to the pot with the cooked lentils.
6. Stir in the lemon zest and lemon juice. Simmer for an additional 5 minutes to allow flavors to blend.
7. Remove from heat and stir in the chopped fresh parsley.
8. Use an immersion blender to blend the soup until smooth, ensuring a liquid consistency suitable for the liquid diet phase.
9. Season with salt to taste.
10. Serve warm.

Nutritional Information (per serving)

- **Total Calories:** 180 kcal
- **Protein:** 12 g
- **Carbohydrates:** 30 g
- **Total Fat:** 1 g
- **Fiber:** 12 g
- **Sodium:** 150 mg

French Onion Soup

Prep Time: 15 minutes | **Cook Time:** 1 hour | **Servings:** 4

Ingredients

- 2 tablespoons olive oil
- 4 large onions, thinly sliced
- 4 cups low-sodium beef broth
- 1/4 cup dry white wine (optional)
- 1 bay leaf
- 1 teaspoon dried thyme
- Salt and pepper to taste
- 4 slices whole grain baguette
- 1/2 cup shredded Gruyere cheese

Instructions

1. In a large pot, heat the olive oil over medium heat. Add the thinly sliced onions and cook, stirring occasionally, until caramelized and golden brown, about 30-40 minutes.
2. Add the low-sodium beef broth, dry white wine (if using), bay leaf, dried thyme, salt, and pepper to the pot with the caramelized onions.
3. Bring the soup to a boil, then reduce the heat to low. Simmer uncovered for 20-30 minutes to allow the flavors to meld.
4. While the soup is simmering, preheat the broiler.
5. Arrange the slices of whole grain baguette on a baking sheet and toast under the broiler until golden brown on both sides.
6. Take out the bay leaf from the soup and discard.
7. Ladle the hot soup into oven-safe bowls. Top each bowl with a slice of toasted whole grain baguette.
8. Sprinkle shredded Gruyere cheese evenly over each slice of baguette.
9. Place the bowls under the broiler for 1-2 minutes, or until the cheese is melted and bubbly.
10. Serve hot.

Nutritional Information (per serving)

- **Total Calories:** 250 kcal
- **Protein:** 12 g
- **Carbohydrates:** 25 g
- **Total Fat:** 10 g
- **Fiber:** 4 g
- **Sodium:** 450 mg

Gazpacho

Prep Time: 15 minutes | **Cook Time:** 0 minutes | **Servings:** 4

Ingredients

- 4 large tomatoes, peeled and chopped
- 1 cucumber, peeled, seeded, and chopped
- 1 red bell pepper, seeded and chopped
- 1/2 red onion, chopped
- 2 cloves garlic, minced
- 2 tablespoons olive oil
- 2 tablespoons red wine vinegar
- 1 tablespoon lemon juice
- 1/2 teaspoon ground cumin
- Salt and pepper to taste
- 1 cup low-sodium vegetable broth
- Optional garnish: chopped fresh parsley or basil

Instructions

1. In a blender or food processor, put together the chopped tomatoes, peeled and chopped cucumber, chopped red bell pepper, chopped red onion, minced garlic, olive oil, red wine vinegar, lemon juice, ground cumin, salt, and pepper.
2. Blend until smooth, adding the low-sodium vegetable broth gradually until desired consistency is achieved for a liquid diet phase.
3. Taste and adjust seasoning as needed.
4. Chill the gazpacho in the refrigerator for at least 1 hour before serving to enhance flavors.
5. Stir adequately before serving and ladle into bowls.
6. Garnish with chopped fresh parsley or basil, if desired.

Nutritional Information (per serving)

- **Total Calories:** 120 kcal
- **Protein:** 3 g
- **Carbohydrates:** 15 g
- **Total Fat:** 6 g
- **Fiber:** 4 g
- **Sodium:** 150 mg

Chapter 4: Pureed Foods Phase

Mashed Sweet Potatoes

Prep Time: 10 minutes | **Cook Time:** 25 minutes | **Number of Servings:** 4

Ingredients:

- 2 large sweet potatoes, peeled and diced
- 1/2 cup low-sodium chicken or vegetable broth
- 1/4 cup plain Greek yogurt
- 1 tablespoon olive oil
- Salt and pepper to taste
- 1/2 teaspoon ground cinnamon (optional)

Instructions:

1. Place the diced sweet potatoes in a large pot and cover with water. Bring to a boil over high heat, then reduce the heat to medium-low and simmer until the sweet potatoes are tender, about 15-20 minutes.
2. Drain the sweet potatoes and return them to the pot. Add the chicken or vegetable broth, Greek yogurt, olive oil, salt, pepper, and cinnamon (if using).
3. Mash the sweet potatoes using a potato masher or fork until smooth and creamy. If needed, you can use a blender or food processor for a finer texture suitable for a pureed diet.
4. Adjust seasoning to taste and serve warm.

Nutritional Information:

- Total Calories: 160 kcal
- Protein: 4 g
- Carbohydrates: 30 g
- Total Fat: 3 g
- Fiber: 4 g
- Sodium: 75 mg

Pureed Carrot and Ginger

Prep Time: 10 minutes | **Cook Time:** 20 minutes | **Number of Servings:** 4

Ingredients:

- 4 large carrots, peeled and sliced
- 1 small onion, chopped
- 1 tablespoon olive oil
- 1 tablespoon grated ginger
- 2 cups low-sodium vegetable broth
- Salt and pepper to taste
- Fresh parsley for garnish (optional)

Instructions:

1. In a large pot, heat olive oil over medium heat. Add chopped onion and sauté until translucent, about 3-4 minutes.
2. Add sliced carrots and grated ginger to the pot. Sauté for an additional 2-3 minutes until fragrant.
3. Pour in the vegetable broth. Bring to a boil, then reduce heat to medium-low. Cover and simmer until the carrots are tender, about 15 minutes.
4. Remove from heat and let it cool slightly.
5. Transfer the mixture to a blender or food processor and puree until smooth. Add more vegetable broth if needed to achieve desired consistency for a pureed diet.
6. Season with salt and pepper to taste.
7. Serve warm, garnished with fresh parsley if desired.

Nutritional Information:

- Total Calories: 90 kcal
- Protein: 2 g
- Carbohydrates: 15 g
- Total Fat: 3 g
- Fiber: 4 g
- Sodium: 80 mg

Creamy Cauliflower Mash

Prep Time: 10 minutes | **Cook Time:** 20 minutes | **Number of Servings:** 4

Ingredients:

- 1 medium head cauliflower, cut into florets
- 2 cloves garlic, minced
- 1/4 cup low-sodium chicken or vegetable broth
- 2 tablespoons plain Greek yogurt
- 1 tablespoon olive oil
- Salt and pepper to taste
- Chopped chives for garnish (optional)

Instructions:

1. Steam or boil the cauliflower florets until very tender, about 10-12 minutes. Drain well.
2. In a small saucepan, heat olive oil over medium heat. Add minced garlic and sauté until fragrant, about 1 minute.
3. Transfer the cooked cauliflower and garlic to a food processor or blender. Add chicken or vegetable broth, Greek yogurt, salt, and pepper.
4. Blend until smooth and creamy, adding more broth if necessary to achieve desired consistency for a pureed diet.
5. Adjust seasoning to taste.
6. Serve warm, garnished with chopped chives if desired.

Nutritional Information:

- Total Calories: 80 kcal
- Protein: 4 g
- Carbohydrates: 10 g
- Total Fat: 3 g
- Fiber: 4 g
- Sodium: 50 mg

Pureed Green Beans with Garlic

Prep Time: 10 minutes | **Cook Time:** 15 minutes | **Number of Servings:** 4

Ingredients:

- 1 pound fresh green beans, trimmed and cut into 1-inch pieces
- 2 cloves garlic, minced
- 1/2 cup low-sodium vegetable broth
- 1 tablespoon olive oil
- Salt and pepper to taste
- Fresh parsley for garnish (optional)

Instructions:

1. Steam or boil the green beans until very tender, about 8-10 minutes. Drain well.
2. In a small saucepan, heat olive oil over medium heat. Add minced garlic and sauté until fragrant, about 1 minute.
3. Add the cooked green beans to the saucepan with the garlic. Stir to coat the green beans with the garlic and olive oil.
4. Add the vegetable broth to the saucepan. Bring to a simmer and cook for an additional 2-3 minutes.
5. Transfer the mixture to a blender or food processor. Blend until smooth, adding more vegetable broth if needed to achieve desired pureed consistency for a bariatric pureed diet.
6. Season with salt and pepper to taste.
7. Serve warm, garnished with fresh parsley if desired.

Nutritional Information:

- Total Calories: 70 kcal
- Protein: 3 g
- Carbohydrates: 10 g
- Total Fat: 3 g
- Fiber: 4 g
- Sodium: 50 mg

Silky Butternut Squash Puree

Prep Time: 10 minutes | **Cook Time:** 30 minutes | **Number of Servings:** 4

Ingredients:

- 1 medium butternut squash, peeled, seeded, and diced
- 1/2 small onion, chopped
- 2 cloves garlic, minced
- 1 tablespoon olive oil
- 1/2 cup low-sodium vegetable broth
- Salt and pepper to taste
- Ground nutmeg for garnish (optional)

Instructions:

1. In a large pot, heat olive oil over medium heat. Add chopped onion and minced garlic. Sauté until onion is translucent, about 3-4 minutes.
2. Add diced butternut squash to the pot. Sauté for an additional 5 minutes, stirring occasionally.
3. Pour in the vegetable broth. Bring to a boil, then reduce heat to medium-low. Cover and simmer until the butternut squash is tender, about 20 minutes.
4. Remove from heat and let it cool slightly.
5. Transfer the mixture to a blender or food processor. Blend until smooth and creamy, adding more vegetable broth if needed to achieve desired pureed consistency for a bariatric pureed diet.
6. Season with salt and pepper to taste.
7. Serve warm, garnished with a sprinkle of ground nutmeg if desired.

Nutritional Information:

- Total Calories: 100 kcal
- Protein: 2 g
- Carbohydrates: 20 g
- Total Fat: 2 g
- Fiber: 4 g
- Sodium: 70 mg

Pureed Peas and Mint

Prep Time: 10 minutes | **Cook Time:** 10 minutes | **Number of Servings:** 4

Ingredients:

- 2 cups frozen peas
- 1/2 small onion, chopped
- 1 clove garlic, minced
- 1 tablespoon olive oil
- 1/2 cup low-sodium vegetable broth
- 1 tablespoon fresh mint leaves, chopped
- Salt and pepper to taste
- Fresh mint leaves for garnish (optional)

Instructions:

1. In a medium saucepan, heat olive oil over medium heat. Add chopped onion and minced garlic. Sauté until onion is translucent, about 3-4 minutes.
2. Add frozen peas to the saucepan. Cook for 2-3 minutes until peas are heated through.
3. Add vegetable broth and chopped mint leaves to the saucepan. Bring to a simmer and cook for an additional 3-4 minutes.
4. Remove from heat and let it cool slightly.
5. Transfer the mixture to a blender or food processor. Blend until smooth and creamy, adding more vegetable broth if needed to achieve desired pureed consistency for a bariatric pureed diet.
6. Season with salt and pepper to taste.
7. Serve warm, garnished with fresh mint leaves if desired.

Nutritional Information:

- Total Calories: 80 kcal
- Protein: 4 g
- Carbohydrates: 12 g
- Total Fat: 2 g
- Fiber: 5 g
- Sodium: 50 mg

Pureed Lentil and Tomato

Prep Time: 10 minutes | **Cook Time:** 30 minutes | **Number of Servings:** 4

Ingredients:

- 1 cup dried green or brown lentils, rinsed
- 1/2 small onion, chopped
- 2 cloves garlic, minced
- 1 tablespoon olive oil
- 1 can (14 oz) diced tomatoes (no salt added)
- 2 cups low-sodium vegetable broth
- 1 teaspoon dried oregano
- Salt and pepper to taste
- Fresh parsley for garnish (optional)

Instructions:

1. In a medium saucepan, heat olive oil over medium heat. Add chopped onion and minced garlic. Sauté until onion is translucent, about 3-4 minutes.
2. Add rinsed lentils, diced tomatoes (including juices), vegetable broth, and dried oregano to the saucepan. Bring to a boil, then reduce heat to low. Cover and simmer until lentils are tender, about 25-30 minutes.
3. Remove from heat and let it cool slightly.
4. Transfer the mixture to a blender or food processor. Blend until smooth and creamy, adding more vegetable broth if needed to achieve desired pureed consistency for a bariatric pureed diet.
5. Season with salt and pepper to taste.
6. Serve warm, garnished with fresh parsley if desired.

Nutritional Information:

- Total Calories: 180 kcal
- Protein: 12 g
- Carbohydrates: 30 g
- Total Fat: 2 g
- Fiber: 12 g
- Sodium: 150 mg

Smooth Apple and Cinnamon

Prep Time: 10 minutes | **Cook Time:** 15 minutes | **Number of Servings:** 4

Ingredients:

- 2 medium apples, peeled, cored, and chopped (use sweet varieties like Gala or Fuji)
- 1/2 teaspoon ground cinnamon
- 1/2 cup low-sodium apple juice or water
- 1 tablespoon chia seeds
- 1 tablespoon almond butter (unsweetened and no added oils)
- Fresh apple slices for garnish (optional)

Instructions:

1. In a medium saucepan, combine chopped apples, ground cinnamon, and apple juice or water.
2. Bring to a boil over medium-high heat. Reduce heat to low, cover, and simmer until apples are very tender, about 10-12 minutes.
3. Remove from heat and let it cool slightly.
4. Transfer the cooked apple mixture to a blender or food processor. Add chia seeds and almond butter.
5. Blend until smooth and creamy, adding more apple juice or water if needed to achieve desired pureed consistency for a bariatric pureed diet.
6. Serve warm or chilled, garnished with fresh apple slices if desired.

Nutritional Information:

- Total Calories: 120 kcal
- Protein: 3 g
- Carbohydrates: 20 g
- Total Fat: 4 g
- Fiber: 5 g
- Sodium: 5 mg

Pureed Chicken and Vegetable

Prep Time: 15 minutes | **Cook Time:** 30 minutes | **Number of Servings:** 4

Ingredients:

- 2 boneless, skinless chicken breasts, diced
- 1 small onion, chopped
- 1 carrot, peeled and chopped
- 1 celery stalk, chopped
- 1 clove garlic, minced
- 1 tablespoon olive oil
- 2 cups low-sodium chicken broth
- 1/2 cup green peas (frozen or fresh)
- 1/2 cup chopped spinach leaves
- Salt and pepper to taste
- Fresh parsley for garnish (optional)

Instructions:

1. In a large saucepan, heat olive oil over medium heat. Add chopped onion, carrot, celery, and minced garlic. Sauté until vegetables are softened, about 5-6 minutes.
2. Add diced chicken breasts to the saucepan. Cook until chicken is no longer pink, about 5-7 minutes.
3. Pour in the chicken broth. Bring to a boil, then reduce heat to low. Cover and simmer until chicken is cooked through and vegetables are tender, about 15 minutes.
4. Stir in green peas and chopped spinach. Cook for an additional 2-3 minutes until peas are heated through and spinach is wilted.
5. Remove from heat and let it cool slightly.
6. Transfer the mixture to a blender or food processor. Blend until smooth and creamy, adding more chicken broth if needed to achieve desired pureed consistency for a bariatric pureed diet.
7. Season with salt and pepper to taste.
8. Serve warm, garnished with fresh parsley if desired.

Nutritional Information:

- Total Calories: 150 kcal
- Protein: 18 g
- Carbohydrates: 8 g
- Total Fat: 5 g
- Fiber: 2 g
- Sodium: 100 mg

Mashed Banana and Avocado

Prep Time: 10 minutes | **Cook Time:** 0 minutes | **Number of Servings:** 2

Ingredients:

- 1 ripe banana
- 1 ripe avocado
- 1 tablespoon almond butter (unsweetened and no added oils)
- 1/2 teaspoon ground cinnamon
- 1/4 teaspoon vanilla extract
- Fresh berries for garnish (optional)

Instructions:

1. Peel and slice the banana and avocado.
2. In a medium bowl, mash the banana and avocado together using a fork or potato masher until smooth.
3. Add almond butter, ground cinnamon, and vanilla extract to the bowl. Mix adequately until all ingredients are combined and the mixture is creamy.
4. Transfer the mixture to a blender or food processor if a smoother texture is desired for the pureed diet phase of a gastric sleeve bariatric diet cookbook.
5. Blend until smooth, adding a small amount of water or almond milk if necessary to achieve desired consistency.
6. Serve chilled or at room temperature, garnished with fresh berries if desired.

Nutritional Information:

- Total Calories: 180 kcal
- Protein: 3 g
- Carbohydrates: 18 g
- Total Fat: 12 g
- Fiber: 7 g
- Sodium: 5 mg

Pureed Turkey with Herbs

Prep Time: 15 minutes | **Cook Time:** 30 minutes | **Number of Servings:** 4

Ingredients:

- 1 pound boneless, skinless turkey breast, diced
- 1/2 small onion, chopped
- 1 carrot, peeled and chopped
- 1 celery stalk, chopped
- 1 clove garlic, minced
- 1 tablespoon olive oil
- 2 cups low-sodium chicken or turkey broth
- 1 teaspoon dried thyme
- 1 teaspoon dried sage
- Salt and pepper to taste
- Fresh parsley for garnish (optional)

Instructions:

1. In a large skillet or saucepan, heat olive oil over medium heat. Add chopped onion, carrot, celery, and minced garlic. Sauté until vegetables are softened, about 5-6 minutes.
2. Add diced turkey breast to the skillet. Cook until turkey is no longer pink, about 5-7 minutes.
3. Pour in the chicken or turkey broth. Bring to a boil, then reduce heat to low. Cover and simmer until turkey is cooked through and vegetables are tender, about 15 minutes.
4. Stir in dried thyme and sage. Cook for an additional 2-3 minutes to allow the flavors to blend.
5. Remove from heat and let it cool slightly.
6. Transfer the mixture to a blender or food processor. Blend until smooth and creamy, adding more broth if needed to achieve desired pureed consistency for a bariatric pureed diet.
7. Season with salt and pepper to taste.
8. Serve warm, garnished with fresh parsley if desired.

Nutritional Information:

- Total Calories: 180 kcal
- Protein: 25 g
- Carbohydrates: 5 g
- Total Fat: 6 g
- Fiber: 1 g
- Sodium: 150 mg

Pureed Black Beans with Cilantro

Prep Time: 10 minutes | **Cook Time:** 20 minutes | **Number of Servings:** 4

Ingredients:

- 1 can (15 oz) black beans, drained and rinsed
- 1/2 small onion, chopped
- 1 clove garlic, minced
- 1 tablespoon olive oil
- 1/4 teaspoon ground cumin
- 1/4 teaspoon ground coriander
- Salt and pepper to taste
- 1/4 cup chopped fresh cilantro
- Fresh lime wedges for garnish (optional)

Instructions:

1. In a medium saucepan, heat olive oil over medium heat. Add chopped onion and minced garlic. Sauté until onions are translucent, about 3-4 minutes.
2. Add drained and rinsed black beans to the saucepan. Stir in ground cumin and ground coriander. Cook for an additional 2-3 minutes to allow the flavors to meld.
3. Add enough water to cover the beans by about 1 inch. Bring to a boil, then reduce heat to low. Cover and simmer for 10 minutes.
4. Remove from heat and let it cool slightly.
5. Transfer the bean mixture to a blender or food processor. Add chopped fresh cilantro.
6. Blend until smooth and creamy, adding more water if needed to achieve desired pureed consistency for a bariatric pureed diet.
7. Season with salt and pepper to taste.
8. Serve warm, garnished with fresh lime wedges if desired.

Nutritional Information:

- Total Calories: 130 kcal
- Protein: 7 g
- Carbohydrates: 20 g
- Total Fat: 3 g
- Fiber: 7 g
- Sodium: 200 mg

Pureed Spinach and Cheese

Prep Time: 10 minutes | **Cook Time:** 10 minutes | **Number of Servings:** 4

Ingredients:

- 8 oz fresh spinach leaves, washed and trimmed
- 1/2 cup low-fat cottage cheese
- 1/4 cup grated Parmesan cheese
- 1 clove garlic, minced
- 1 tablespoon olive oil
- Salt and pepper to taste
- Pinch of nutmeg (optional)

Instructions:

1. In a large skillet or saucepan, heat olive oil over medium heat. Add minced garlic and sauté until fragrant, about 1 minute.
2. Add fresh spinach leaves to the skillet. Cook, stirring frequently, until spinach is wilted and tender, about 3-4 minutes.
3. Remove spinach from heat and let it cool slightly.
4. In a blender or food processor, combine cooked spinach, low-fat cottage cheese, grated Parmesan cheese, and a pinch of nutmeg if using.
5. Blend until smooth, adding a small amount of water if necessary to achieve desired pureed consistency for a bariatric pureed diet.
6. Season with salt and pepper to taste.
7. Serve warm, adjusting seasoning if needed.

Nutritional Information:

- Total Calories: 90 kcal
- Protein: 9 g
- Carbohydrates: 4 g
- Total Fat: 4 g
- Fiber: 2 g
- Sodium: 150 mg

Pureed Zucchini and Basil

Prep Time: 10 minutes | **Cook Time:** 10 minutes | **Number of Servings:** 4

Ingredients:

- 2 medium zucchini, sliced
- 1/4 cup fresh basil leaves
- 1 clove garlic, minced
- 1 tablespoon olive oil
- Salt and pepper to taste
- Water, as needed for blending

Instructions:

1. In a large skillet, heat olive oil over medium heat. Add minced garlic and sauté for about 1 minute until fragrant.
2. Add sliced zucchini to the skillet. Cook, stirring occasionally, until zucchini is tender, about 5-7 minutes.
3. Remove skillet from heat and let the zucchini cool slightly.
4. In a blender or food processor, combine cooked zucchini, fresh basil leaves, and a pinch of salt and pepper.
5. Blend until smooth, adding water gradually as needed to achieve a smooth pureed consistency suitable for a bariatric pureed diet.
6. Adjust seasoning if necessary.
7. Serve warm.

Nutritional Information:

- Total Calories: 50 kcal
- Protein: 2 g
- Carbohydrates: 5 g
- Total Fat: 3 g
- Fiber: 2 g
- Sodium: 10 mg

Smooth Mango and Yogurt

Prep Time: 10 minutes | **Cook Time:** 0 minutes | **Number of Servings:** 2

Ingredients:

- 1 cup ripe mango, peeled and diced
- 1/2 cup plain Greek yogurt
- 1/4 teaspoon vanilla extract
- 1 tablespoon chia seeds (optional for added fiber)

Instructions:

1. In a blender, combine diced mango, Greek yogurt, vanilla extract, and chia seeds (if using).
2. Blend until smooth and creamy, adding a small amount of water if needed to achieve desired consistency for a pureed diet.
3. Pour into serving glasses.
4. Serve chilled.

Nutritional Information:

- Total Calories: 120 kcal
- Protein: 6 g
- Carbohydrates: 20 g
- Total Fat: 1 g
- Fiber: 3 g
- Sodium: 25 mg

Mashed Pumpkin with Spices

Prep Time: 10 minutes | **Cook Time:** 20 minutes | **Number of Servings:** 4

Ingredients:

- 1 small pumpkin (about 2 pounds), peeled, seeded, and cut into chunks
- 1/2 teaspoon ground cinnamon
- 1/4 teaspoon ground nutmeg
- 1/4 teaspoon ground ginger
- Salt, to taste
- Pepper, to taste

Instructions:

1. In a large pot, bring water to a boil. Add the pumpkin chunks and cook until tender, about 15-20 minutes.
2. Drain the cooked pumpkin and transfer to a food processor or blender.
3. Add ground cinnamon, ground nutmeg, ground ginger, salt, and pepper to the pumpkin.
4. Puree until smooth and creamy, adding a small amount of water if needed to achieve desired consistency for a pureed diet.
5. Adjust seasoning if necessary.
6. Serve warm.

Nutritional Information:

- Total Calories: 70 kcal
- Protein: 2 g
- Carbohydrates: 17 g
- Total Fat: 0.5 g
- Fiber: 3 g
- Sodium: 5 mg

Pureed Beets with Orange

Prep Time: 10 minutes | **Cook Time:** 45 minutes | **Number of Servings:** 4

Ingredients:

- 4 medium beets, peeled and diced
- 1 orange, juiced and zested
- 1 tablespoon olive oil
- Salt, to taste
- Pepper, to taste

Instructions:

1. In a medium pot, add the diced beets and cover with water. Bring to a boil over medium-high heat, then reduce the heat and simmer until the beets are tender, about 30-40 minutes.
2. Drain the cooked beets and transfer to a food processor or blender.
3. Add the orange juice, orange zest, olive oil, salt, and pepper to the beets.
4. Puree until smooth, adding a small amount of water if needed to achieve desired consistency for a pureed diet.
5. Adjust seasoning if necessary.
6. Serve warm or chilled.

Nutritional Information:

- Total Calories: 80 kcal
- Protein: 2 g
- Carbohydrates: 15 g
- Total Fat: 2 g
- Fiber: 4 g
- Sodium: 80 mg

Pureed Cauliflower and Cheese

Prep Time: 10 minutes | **Cook Time:** 20 minutes | **Number of Servings:** 4

Ingredients:

- 1 medium head cauliflower, cut into florets
- 1 cup low-fat cottage cheese
- 1/2 cup grated Parmesan cheese
- 1/4 teaspoon garlic powder
- Salt, to taste
- Pepper, to taste

Instructions:

1. Steam or boil the cauliflower florets until very tender, about 10-12 minutes.
2. Drain the cauliflower well and transfer to a food processor or blender.
3. Add the cottage cheese, Parmesan cheese, garlic powder, salt, and pepper to the cauliflower.
4. Puree until smooth, adding a small amount of water if needed to achieve desired consistency for a pureed diet.
5. Adjust seasoning if necessary.
6. Serve warm.

Nutritional Information:

- Total Calories: 120 kcal
- Protein: 12 g
- Carbohydrates: 10 g
- Total Fat: 4 g
- Fiber: 4 g
- Sodium: 300 mg

Pureed Lentil and Spinach

Prep Time: 10 minutes | **Cook Time:** 30 minutes | **Number of Servings:** 4

Ingredients:

- 1 cup dried green or brown lentils, rinsed
- 1/2 small onion, chopped
- 2 cloves garlic, minced
- 1 tablespoon olive oil
- 4 cups fresh spinach leaves
- 3 cups low-sodium vegetable broth
- 1 teaspoon ground cumin
- Salt and pepper, to taste

Instructions:

1. In a medium saucepan, heat olive oil over medium heat. Add chopped onion and minced garlic. Sauté until the onion is translucent, about 3-4 minutes.
2. Add rinsed lentils and ground cumin to the saucepan. Stir to combine.
3. Pour in the low-sodium vegetable broth. Bring to a boil, then reduce heat to low. Cover and simmer until the lentils are tender, about 20-25 minutes.
4. Add fresh spinach leaves to the saucepan. Cook for an additional 2-3 minutes, until the spinach is wilted.
5. Remove from heat and let the mixture cool slightly.
6. Transfer the mixture to a blender or food processor. Puree until smooth, adding more broth if needed to achieve the desired consistency for a pureed diet.
7. Season with salt and pepper to taste.
8. Serve warm.

Nutritional Information:

- Total Calories: 150 kcal
- Protein: 10 g
- Carbohydrates: 22 g
- Total Fat: 3 g
- Fiber: 8 g
- Sodium: 100 mg

Pureed Sweet Potato and Coconut

Prep Time: 10 minutes | **Cook Time:** 20 minutes | **Number of Servings:** 4

Ingredients:

- 2 medium sweet potatoes, peeled and diced
- 1/2 cup light coconut milk
- 1/2 teaspoon ground cinnamon
- 1/4 teaspoon ground ginger
- 1 tablespoon olive oil
- Salt, to taste
- Fresh cilantro for garnish (optional)

Instructions:

1. In a large pot, bring water to a boil. Add the diced sweet potatoes and cook until tender, about 15 minutes.
2. Drain the cooked sweet potatoes and transfer them to a food processor or blender.
3. Add light coconut milk, ground cinnamon, ground ginger, and olive oil to the sweet potatoes.
4. Puree until smooth and creamy, adding a small amount of water if needed to achieve desired consistency for a pureed diet.
5. Season with salt to taste.
6. Serve warm, garnished with fresh cilantro if desired.

Nutritional Information:

- Total Calories: 120 kcal
- Protein: 2 g
- Carbohydrates: 24 g
- Total Fat: 3 g
- Fiber: 4 g
- Sodium: 20 mg

Mashed Pear and Ginger

Prep Time: 10 minutes | **Cook Time:** 15 minutes | **Number of Servings:** 4

Ingredients:

- 4 medium pears, peeled, cored, and diced
- 1 teaspoon fresh ginger, grated
- 1 tablespoon lemon juice
- 1/4 cup water
- 1/4 teaspoon ground cinnamon
- Salt, to taste

Instructions:

1. In a medium saucepan, combine diced pears, grated ginger, lemon juice, and water.
2. Bring the mixture to a boil over medium-high heat. Reduce heat to low, cover, and simmer until pears are very tender, about 10-12 minutes.
3. Remove from heat and let it cool slightly.
4. Transfer the mixture to a blender or food processor. Add ground cinnamon and a pinch of salt.
5. Puree until smooth, adding more water if needed to achieve desired consistency for a pureed diet.
6. Adjust seasoning if necessary.
7. Serve warm or chilled.

Nutritional Information:

- Total Calories: 60 kcal
- Protein: 0.5 g
- Carbohydrates: 16 g
- Total Fat: 0 g
- Fiber: 4 g
- Sodium: 2 mg

Pureed Eggplant and Garlic

Prep Time: 10 minutes | **Cook Time:** 30 minutes | **Number of Servings:** 4

Ingredients:

- 1 large eggplant, peeled and diced
- 2 cloves garlic, minced
- 1 tablespoon olive oil
- 1/4 teaspoon ground cumin
- 1/4 teaspoon ground coriander
- Salt, to taste
- Pepper, to taste

Instructions:

1. Preheat the oven to 400°F (200°C).
2. Place the diced eggplant on a baking sheet. Drizzle with olive oil and sprinkle with minced garlic, ground cumin, and ground coriander. Toss to coat evenly.
3. Roast in the preheated oven for 20-25 minutes, until the eggplant is tender and golden brown.
4. Remove from the oven and let it cool slightly.
5. Transfer the roasted eggplant and garlic to a blender or food processor. Blend until smooth, adding a small amount of water if needed to achieve desired consistency for a pureed diet.
6. Season with salt and pepper to taste.
7. Serve warm or chilled.

Nutritional Information:

- Total Calories: 70 kcal
- Protein: 1 g
- Carbohydrates: 9 g
- Total Fat: 4 g
- Fiber: 3 g
- Sodium: 5 mg

Pureed Tomato and Basil

Prep Time: 10 minutes | **Cook Time:** 20 minutes | **Number of Servings:** 4

Ingredients:

- 4 large tomatoes, peeled and diced
- 1/2 small onion, chopped
- 2 cloves garlic, minced
- 1 tablespoon olive oil
- 1/4 cup fresh basil leaves, chopped
- Salt, to taste
- Pepper, to taste

Instructions:

1. In a large saucepan, heat olive oil over medium heat. Add chopped onion and minced garlic. Sauté until the onion is translucent, about 5 minutes.
2. Add diced tomatoes to the saucepan. Cook for 10-15 minutes, until the tomatoes are soft and the flavors are well combined.
3. Remove from heat and let the mixture cool slightly.
4. Transfer the tomato mixture to a blender or food processor. Add chopped fresh basil leaves.
5. Blend until smooth, adding a small amount of water if needed to achieve desired consistency for a pureed diet.
6. Season with salt and pepper to taste.
7. Serve warm.

Nutritional Information:

- Total Calories: 70 kcal
- Protein: 2 g
- Carbohydrates: 8 g
- Total Fat: 4 g
- Fiber: 2 g
- Sodium: 10 mg

Pureed Squash and Sage

Prep Time: 10 minutes | **Cook Time:** 25 minutes | **Number of Servings:** 4

Ingredients:

- 1 medium butternut squash, peeled, seeded, and diced
- 1 tablespoon olive oil
- 1/2 teaspoon dried sage
- Salt, to taste
- Pepper, to taste
- Water or low-sodium vegetable broth, as needed for blending

Instructions:

1. In a large pot, bring water to a boil. Add the diced butternut squash and cook until tender, about 15-20 minutes.
2. Drain the cooked squash and transfer to a blender or food processor.
3. Add olive oil, dried sage, salt, and pepper to the squash.
4. Puree until smooth, adding a small amount of water or low-sodium vegetable broth if needed to achieve desired consistency for a pureed diet.
5. Adjust seasoning if necessary.
6. Serve warm.

Nutritional Information:

- Total Calories: 90 kcal
- Protein: 1.5 g

Chapter 5: Soft Foods Phase

Soft Scrambled Eggs

Prep Time: 5 minutes | **Cook Time:** 5 minutes | **Servings:** 1

Ingredients:

- 2 large eggs
- 1 tablespoon low-fat milk
- Salt and pepper to taste
- 1 teaspoon olive oil
- 1/4 cup diced bell peppers (any color)
- 1/4 cup diced tomatoes
- 1 tablespoon chopped fresh parsley (optional)

Instructions:

1. Crack the eggs into a bowl, add the milk, salt, and pepper. Whisk until well combined.
2. Heat the olive oil in a non-stick skillet over medium heat.
3. Add the diced bell peppers and tomatoes to the skillet. Cook for 2-3 minutes until softened.
4. Pour the egg mixture into the skillet. Let it sit for a few seconds until the edges start to set.
5. Using a spatula, gently push the eggs from the edges towards the center of the skillet. Continue this process, gently folding the eggs over themselves, until they are softly scrambled and no liquid egg remains.
6. Remove from heat immediately once the eggs are cooked but still moist. Stir in chopped parsley if desired.

Nutritional Information:

- **Total Calories:** 210 kcal
- **Protein:** 17g
- **Carbohydrates:** 7g
- **Total Fat:** 12g
- **Fiber:** 2g
- **Sodium:** 320mg

Cottage Cheese with Pineapple

Prep Time: 5 minutes | **Cook Time:** 0 minutes | **Servings:** 1

Ingredients:

- 1/2 cup low-fat cottage cheese
- 1/2 cup diced fresh pineapple
- 1 tablespoon chopped walnuts (optional)
- 1 teaspoon honey or agave syrup (optional, for sweetness)

Instructions:

1. If using honey or agave syrup, drizzle it over the diced pineapple and toss gently to coat.
2. In a serving bowl, layer the low-fat cottage cheese.
3. Top with the diced pineapple (with or without honey/agave syrup).
4. Sprinkle chopped walnuts on top for added texture and healthy fats.
5. Enjoy immediately as a soft and nutritious snack or meal option.

Nutritional Information:

- **Total Calories:** 220 kcal
- **Protein:** 18g
- **Carbohydrates:** 26g
- **Total Fat:** 4g
- **Fiber:** 3g
- **Sodium:** 180mg

Soft Poached Salmon

Prep Time: 5 minutes | **Cook Time:** 10 minutes | **Servings:** 1

Ingredients:

- 1 piece of salmon fillet (about 4 oz)
- 1 cup low-sodium vegetable broth
- 1/2 lemon, sliced
- 1/4 teaspoon dried dill (optional)
- Salt and pepper to taste

Instructions:

1. In a small saucepan, pour the vegetable broth and add the sliced lemon and dried dill. Bring to a gentle simmer over medium heat.
2. Carefully add the salmon fillet to the simmering broth. The broth should just cover the fish. If needed, add more broth or water.
3. Reduce heat to low and cover the saucepan. Let the salmon poach gently for about 8-10 minutes, depending on thickness, until the fish is opaque and flakes easily with a fork.
4. Take out the poached salmon from the broth using a slotted spoon, being gentle to keep it intact.
5. Season with salt and pepper to taste.
6. Serve immediately while warm and soft.

Nutritional Information:

- **Total Calories:** 250 kcal
- **Protein:** 28g
- **Carbohydrates:** 2g
- **Total Fat:** 14g
- **Fiber:** 0g
- **Sodium:** 180mg

Greek Yogurt with Honey

Prep Time: 2 minutes | **Cook Time:** 0 minutes | **Servings:** 1

Ingredients:

- 1/2 cup plain Greek yogurt (low-fat or non-fat)
- 1 teaspoon honey
- 1 tablespoon chopped nuts (such as almonds or walnuts) (optional)
- Fresh berries (optional, for garnish)

Instructions:

1. In a small bowl, scoop the Greek yogurt.
2. Drizzle the honey over the Greek yogurt.
3. Sprinkle chopped nuts on top for added texture and healthy fats.
4. Add fresh berries for extra flavor and fiber.
5. Enjoy immediately as a soft and nutritious snack or meal option.

Nutritional Information:

- **Total Calories:** 160 kcal
- **Protein:** 15g
- **Carbohydrates:** 20g
- **Total Fat:** 2g
- **Fiber:** 1g
- **Sodium:** 40mg

Mashed Avocado with Lime

Prep Time: 5 minutes | **Cook Time:** 0 minutes | **Servings:** 1

Ingredients:

- 1 ripe avocado
- Juice of 1/2 lime
- Salt and pepper to taste

Instructions:

1. Cut the avocado in half, take out the pit, and scoop out the flesh into a bowl.
2. Using a fork, mash the avocado until smooth and creamy.
3. Squeeze the juice of half a lime over the mashed avocado.
4. Add salt and pepper to taste.
5. Stir adequately to combine all ingredients evenly.
6. Enjoy immediately as a soft and nutritious snack or meal option.

Nutritional Information:

- **Total Calories:** 160 kcal
- **Protein:** 2g
- **Carbohydrates:** 9g
- **Total Fat:** 14g
- **Fiber:** 7g
- **Sodium:** 5mg

Soft Boiled Eggs

Prep Time: 2 minutes | **Cook Time:** 6 minutes | **Servings:** 1

Ingredients:

- 2 large eggs

Instructions:

1. Bring a small pot of water to a boil over medium-high heat.
2. Gently lower the eggs into the boiling water using a spoon.
3. Boil the eggs for exactly 6 minutes for a soft-boiled texture.
4. Immediately take out the eggs from the boiling water and place them into a bowl of ice water to stop the cooking process.
5. Once cooled, carefully peel the eggs.
6. Serve the soft-boiled eggs immediately while warm and soft.

Nutritional Information:

- **Total Calories:** 140 kcal
- **Protein:** 12g
- **Carbohydrates:** 1g
- **Total Fat:** 10g
- **Fiber:** 0g
- **Sodium:** 140mg

Tuna Salad with Yogurt

Prep Time: 10 minutes | **Cook Time:** 0 minutes | **Servings:** 1

Ingredients:

- 1 small can (about 5 oz) tuna in water, drained
- 1/4 cup plain Greek yogurt (low-fat or non-fat)
- 1/4 cup diced cucumber
- 1/4 cup diced red bell pepper
- 1 tablespoon chopped fresh parsley (optional)
- Salt and pepper to taste

Instructions:

1. In a mixing bowl, put together the drained tuna, plain Greek yogurt, diced cucumber, diced red bell pepper, and chopped fresh parsley.
2. Stir gently until all ingredients are well combined.
3. Season with salt and pepper to taste.
4. Enjoy the tuna salad immediately as a soft and nutritious meal option.

Nutritional Information:

- **Total Calories:** 220 kcal
- **Protein:** 30g
- **Carbohydrates:** 9g
- **Total Fat:** 6g
- **Fiber:** 2g
- **Sodium:** 180mg

Soft Baked Apple with Cinnamon

Prep Time: 5 minutes | **Cook Time:** 20 minutes | **Servings:** 1

Ingredients:

- 1 medium apple (such as Gala or Fuji)
- 1/2 teaspoon ground cinnamon
- 1 teaspoon honey (optional, omit if avoiding simple sugars)
- 1 tablespoon chopped nuts (such as almonds or walnuts) (optional)

Instructions:

1. Preheat the oven to 350°F (175°C).
2. Core the apple using an apple corer or a knife, leaving the bottom intact. Place the apple upright in a small baking dish.
3. Sprinkle the ground cinnamon evenly over the apple.
4. Drizzle honey over the apple if using.
5. Bake the apple in the preheated oven for about 20 minutes, or until the apple is tender and can be easily pierced with a fork.
6. If desired, sprinkle chopped nuts over the baked apple for added texture and healthy fats.
7. Enjoy the soft baked apple warm, either plain or with a dollop of Greek yogurt for extra protein.

Nutritional Information:

- **Total Calories:** 150 kcal
- **Protein:** 2g
- **Carbohydrates:** 30g
- **Total Fat:** 3g
- **Fiber:** 5g
- **Sodium:** 0mg

Soft Tofu with Soy Sauce

Prep Time: 5 minutes | **Cook Time:** 5 minutes | **Servings:** 1

Ingredients:

- 1/2 block (about 150g) soft tofu
- 1 tablespoon low-sodium soy sauce
- 1/2 teaspoon sesame oil
- 1 green onion, finely chopped
- 1 teaspoon sesame seeds (optional, for garnish)

Instructions:

1. Cut the soft tofu into bite-sized cubes.
2. Heat a small non-stick skillet over medium heat.
3. Add the tofu cubes to the skillet and cook gently for about 3-4 minutes, stirring occasionally, until heated through.
4. In a small bowl, mix together the low-sodium soy sauce and sesame oil.
5. Pour the soy sauce mixture over the cooked tofu in the skillet. Gently stir to coat the tofu evenly with the sauce.
6. Cook for an additional 1-2 minutes until the sauce is warmed through and slightly thickened.
7. Remove from heat and sprinkle with chopped green onions and sesame seeds if using.
8. Transfer the soft tofu with soy sauce to a plate and enjoy warm.

Nutritional Information:

- **Total Calories:** 150 kcal
- **Protein:** 12g
- **Carbohydrates:** 7g
- **Total Fat:** 8g
- **Fiber:** 1g
- **Sodium:** 300mg

Soft Cooked Oatmeal

Prep Time: 2 minutes | **Cook Time:** 5 minutes | **Servings:** 1

Ingredients:

- 1/2 cup old-fashioned oats
- 1 cup water
- Pinch of salt
- 1/4 cup unsweetened almond milk (optional, for added creaminess)
- 1 tablespoon ground flaxseed (optional, for added fiber and healthy fats)
- Fresh berries or sliced banana (optional, for garnish)

Instructions:

1. In a small saucepan, bring the water to a boil over medium-high heat.
2. Add the old-fashioned oats and a pinch of salt to the boiling water.
3. Reduce the heat to low and simmer the oats for about 5 minutes, stirring occasionally, until the oats are soft and the mixture has thickened to your desired consistency.
4. If using, stir in the unsweetened almond milk and ground flaxseed to the cooked oatmeal for added creaminess, fiber, and healthy fats.
5. Take out the soft cooked oatmeal from the heat and transfer to a bowl.
6. Garnish with fresh berries or sliced banana if desired.

Nutritional Information:

- **Total Calories:** 200 kcal
- **Protein:** 7g
- **Carbohydrates:** 33g
- **Total Fat:** 5g
- **Fiber:** 5g
- **Sodium:** 50mg

Mashed Banana with Yogurt

Prep Time: 5 minutes | **Cook Time:** 0 minutes | **Servings:** 1

Ingredients:

- 1 ripe banana
- 1/2 cup plain Greek yogurt (low-fat or non-fat)
- Cinnamon or nutmeg for garnish (optional)

Instructions:

1. Peel the ripe banana and place it in a small mixing bowl.
2. Using a fork, mash the banana until smooth and creamy.
3. Add the plain Greek yogurt to the mashed banana. Stir adequately until fully combined.
4. Sprinkle with cinnamon or nutmeg if desired for additional flavor.
5. Enjoy the mashed banana with yogurt immediately as a soft and nutritious snack or meal option.

Nutritional Information:

- **Total Calories:** 160 kcal
- **Protein:** 14g
- **Carbohydrates:** 30g
- **Total Fat:** 0.5g
- **Fiber:** 3g
- **Sodium:** 35mg

Soft Baked Sweet Potato

Prep Time: 5 minutes | **Cook Time:** 45 minutes | **Servings:** 1

Ingredients:

- 1 small sweet potato

Instructions:

1. Preheat the oven to 400°F (200°C).
2. Wash the sweet potato thoroughly under cold water and pat dry with a paper towel.
3. Pierce the sweet potato several times with a fork or knife to allow steam to escape during baking.
4. Place the sweet potato directly on the oven rack or on a baking sheet lined with aluminum foil.
5. Bake the sweet potato for 45-50 minutes, or until it is very tender when pierced with a fork. The skin should be wrinkled and the inside soft.
6. Take out the sweet potato from the oven and allow it to cool slightly.
7. Cut the sweet potato open lengthwise and fluff the flesh with a fork.
8. Serve immediately as is, or with a sprinkle of cinnamon or a drizzle of olive oil for added flavor.

Nutritional Information:

- **Total Calories:** 120 kcal
- **Protein:** 2g
- **Carbohydrates:** 27g
- **Total Fat:** 0.2g
- **Fiber:** 4g
- **Sodium:** 20mg

Soft Roasted Squash

Prep Time: 10 minutes | **Cook Time:** 45 minutes | **Servings:** 2

Ingredients:

- 1 small butternut squash
- 1 tablespoon olive oil
- Salt and pepper, to taste
- Fresh herbs (optional, for garnish)

Instructions:

1. Preheat the oven to 400°F (200°C).
2. Wash the butternut squash thoroughly. Peel the squash using a vegetable peeler. Cut the squash in half lengthwise and scoop out the seeds with a spoon. Cut into cubes.
3. Place the cubed squash on a baking sheet lined with parchment paper.
4. Drizzle olive oil over the squash cubes, season with salt and pepper to taste, and toss gently to coat evenly.
5. Roast the squash in the preheated oven for 40-45 minutes, or until the squash is tender and lightly caramelized, stirring halfway through cooking.
6. Remove from the oven and let cool slightly.
7. Garnish with fresh herbs if desired, such as parsley or thyme.

Nutritional Information:

- **Total Calories:** 120 kcal
- **Protein:** 2g
- **Carbohydrates:** 20g
- **Total Fat:** 5g
- **Fiber:** 4g
- **Sodium:** 5mg

Cottage Cheese with Tomato

Prep Time: 5 minutes | **Cook Time:** 0 minutes | **Servings:** 1

Ingredients:

- 1/2 cup low-fat cottage cheese
- 1 small tomato, diced
- Fresh basil leaves, chopped, for garnish (optional)
- Salt and pepper, to taste

Instructions:

1. Dice the tomato into small pieces.
2. If desired, chop fresh basil leaves for garnish.
3. In a serving bowl, place the cottage cheese.
4. Top with diced tomato pieces.
5. Season with salt and pepper to taste.
6. Garnish with chopped basil leaves, if using.

Nutritional Information:

- **Total Calories:** 120 kcal
- **Protein:** 14g
- **Carbohydrates:** 8g
- **Total Fat:** 3g
- **Fiber:** 1g
- **Sodium:** 280mg

Soft Cooked Lentils

Prep Time: 5 minutes | **Cook Time:** 20 minutes | **Servings:** 2

Ingredients:

- 1/2 cup dry brown or green lentils
- 1 1/2 cups water
- Salt, to taste

Instructions:

1. Rinse the lentils under cold water and drain.
2. In a medium saucepan, put together the rinsed lentils and water.
3. Bring to a boil over high heat.
4. Reduce the heat to low, cover the saucepan, and simmer gently for 15-20 minutes, or until the lentils are tender and cooked through. Stir occasionally.
5. Add salt to taste during the last few minutes of cooking, if desired.
6. Once cooked, drain any excess water if necessary.
7. Serve the soft cooked lentils warm.

Nutritional Information:

- **Total Calories:** 160 kcal
- **Protein:** 12g
- **Carbohydrates:** 28g
- **Total Fat:** 1g
- **Fiber:** 12g
- **Sodium:** 5mg

Soft Steamed Broccoli

Prep Time: 5 minutes | **Cook Time:** 5 minutes | **Servings:** 2

Ingredients:

- 1 head of broccoli, cut into florets

Instructions:

1. Cut the broccoli into small florets.
2. Place the broccoli florets in a steamer basket over boiling water.
3. Steam the broccoli for about 5 minutes, or until tender. Ensure that the broccoli is soft and easily pierced with a fork.
4. Once steamed, take out the broccoli from the steamer basket.
5. Serve the soft steamed broccoli warm.

Nutritional Information:

- **Total Calories:** 50 kcal
- **Protein:** 4g
- **Carbohydrates:** 10g
- **Total Fat:** 0.5g
- **Fiber:** 5g
- **Sodium:** 30mg

Soft Baked Pear with Nutmeg

Prep Time: 10 minutes | **Cook Time:** 30 minutes | **Servings:** 2

Ingredients:

- 2 ripe pears, peeled, cored, and sliced
- 1/2 teaspoon ground nutmeg
- 1 tablespoon honey (optional, for sweetness)

Instructions:

1. Preheat the oven to 350°F (175°C).
2. Peel, core, and slice the pears into thin slices.
3. Arrange the pear slices in a baking dish.
4. Sprinkle the ground nutmeg evenly over the pear slices.
5. Optionally, drizzle honey over the pears for added sweetness.
6. Cover the baking dish with foil or a lid.
7. Bake in the preheated oven for about 30 minutes, or until the pears are soft and tender.
8. Remove from the oven and let cool slightly.
9. Serve the soft baked pears warm, either alone or with a dollop of Greek yogurt.

Nutritional Information:

- **Total Calories:** 120 kcal
- **Protein:** 1g
- **Carbohydrates:** 30g
- **Total Fat:** 0.5g
- **Fiber:** 6g
- **Sodium:** 0mg

Soft Tofu Scramble

Prep Time: 10 minutes | **Cook Time:** 10 minutes | **Servings:** 2

Ingredients:

- 200g soft tofu, crumbled
- 1/2 small onion, finely chopped
- 1/2 red bell pepper, finely diced
- 1/2 cup spinach leaves, chopped
- 1 garlic clove, minced
- 1/2 teaspoon turmeric powder
- Salt and pepper to taste
- 1 tablespoon olive oil

Instructions:

1. Crumble the soft tofu into small pieces and set aside.
2. Finely chop the onion, dice the red bell pepper, chop the spinach, and mince the garlic.
3. Heat olive oil in a non-stick skillet over medium heat.
4. Add the chopped onion and cook until softened, about 3 minutes.
5. Add the diced red bell pepper and minced garlic to the skillet. Cook for an additional 2 minutes until the peppers are tender.
6. Sprinkle turmeric powder over the vegetables and stir adequately to combine, cooking for 1 minute until fragrant.
7. Add the crumbled tofu to the skillet, gently stirring to combine with the vegetables.
8. Cook the tofu mixture for about 3-4 minutes, stirring occasionally, until heated through.
9. Season with salt and pepper to taste.
10. Serve the soft tofu scramble warm, optionally garnished with chopped parsley or chives.

Nutritional Information:

- **Total Calories:** 150 kcal
- **Protein:** 12g
- **Carbohydrates:** 8g
- **Total Fat:** 8g
- **Fiber:** 3g
- **Sodium:** 150mg

Soft Baked Fish with Herbs

Prep Time: 10 minutes | **Cook Time:** 20 minutes | **Servings:** 2

Ingredients:

- 2 fillets of white fish (such as tilapia or cod), about 200g each
- 1 tablespoon olive oil
- 1 tablespoon fresh parsley, finely chopped
- 1 tablespoon fresh dill, finely chopped
- 1 garlic clove, minced
- Salt and pepper to taste
- Lemon wedges for serving

Instructions:

1. Preheat the oven to 375°F (190°C).
2. Pat dry the fish fillets with paper towels and place them in a baking dish.
3. In a small bowl, put together the olive oil, chopped parsley, chopped dill, minced garlic, salt, and pepper.
4. Brush the herb mixture evenly over the fish fillets, coating both sides.
5. Cover the baking dish with foil and bake in the preheated oven for about 15-20 minutes, or until the fish is opaque and flakes easily with a fork.
6. Remove from the oven and serve the soft baked fish immediately, garnished with lemon wedges.

Nutritional Information:

- **Total Calories:** 200 kcal
- **Protein:** 25g
- **Carbohydrates:** 2g
- **Total Fat:** 10g
- **Fiber:** 0.5g
- **Sodium:** 70mg

Soft Cooked Quinoa

Prep Time: 5 minutes | **Cook Time:** 15 minutes | **Servings:** 2

Ingredients:

- 1/2 cup quinoa
- 1 cup water or low-sodium vegetable broth

Instructions:

1. Rinse the quinoa thoroughly under cold water in a fine-mesh sieve.
2. In a small saucepan, put together the rinsed quinoa and water or vegetable broth. Bring to a boil over medium-high heat.
3. Reduce the heat to low, cover with a lid, and simmer for 15 minutes, or until the quinoa is tender and all the liquid is absorbed.
4. Take out the saucepan from heat and let it sit, covered, for 5 minutes. Fluff the quinoa gently with a fork.
5. Serve the soft cooked quinoa warm as desired.

Nutritional Information:

- **Total Calories:** 110 kcal
- **Protein:** 4g
- **Carbohydrates:** 20g
- **Total Fat:** 1.5g
- **Fiber:** 2.5g
- **Sodium:** 5mg

Soft Steamed Green Beans

Prep Time: 10 minutes | **Cook Time:** 10 minutes | **Servings:** 2

Ingredients:

- 1/2 lb fresh green beans, ends trimmed
- Water for steaming

Instructions:

1. Wash the green beans thoroughly under cold water. Trim the ends if necessary.
2. Fill a pot with a few inches of water and bring it to a boil over medium-high heat. Place a steamer basket or colander over the pot.
3. Add the prepared green beans to the steamer basket or colander. Cover with a lid and steam for about 8-10 minutes, or until the green beans are tender.
4. Check the green beans periodically for doneness by piercing with a fork. They should be tender but still retain their shape.
5. Take out the green beans from the steamer and transfer to a serving dish. Serve warm.

Nutritional Information:

- **Total Calories:** 30 kcal
- **Protein:** 2g
- **Carbohydrates:** 7g
- **Total Fat:** 0g
- **Fiber:** 3g
- **Sodium:** 5mg

Soft Baked Potato with Cheese

Prep Time: 10 minutes | **Cook Time:** 1 hour | **Servings:** 2

Ingredients:

- 2 medium russet potatoes
- 1/4 cup shredded low-fat cheddar cheese
- Salt (optional, to taste)
- Freshly ground black pepper (optional, to taste)

Instructions:

1. Preheat the oven to 400°F (200°C).
2. Scrub the potatoes thoroughly under cold water to remove any dirt. Pat dry with a clean towel.
3. Pierce each potato several times with a fork or knife. This allows steam to escape during baking.
4. Place the potatoes directly on the oven rack and bake for about 1 hour, or until tender when pierced with a fork. The skin should be crisp.
5. Take out the potatoes from the oven. Using a knife, cut each potato in half lengthwise.
6. Gently scoop out some of the flesh from each potato half, leaving a thin layer attached to the skin to create a shell.
7. Mash the scooped potato flesh with a fork in a bowl until smooth.
8. Fold in the shredded cheese into the mashed potato until well combined.
9. Spoon the mashed potato and cheese mixture back into the potato shells, dividing evenly.
10. Place the filled potato halves back on the baking sheet and return to the oven for an additional 5-10 minutes, or until the cheese is melted and bubbly.
11. Remove from the oven and season with salt and pepper if desired.
12. Serve immediately while warm.

Nutritional Information:

- **Total Calories:** 230 kcal
- **Protein:** 10g
- **Carbohydrates:** 45g
- **Total Fat:** 1g
- **Fiber:** 4g
- **Sodium:** 75mg

Soft Roasted Beet Salad

Prep Time: 10 minutes | **Cook Time:** 1 hour | **Servings:** 2

Ingredients:

- 2 medium beets, peeled and diced
- 1 tablespoon olive oil
- Salt, to taste
- Freshly ground black pepper, to taste
- 1/4 cup crumbled feta cheese
- 2 cups baby spinach leaves
- 1/4 cup chopped walnuts, toasted

Instructions:

1. Preheat the oven to 400°F (200°C).
2. Place the diced beets on a baking sheet. Drizzle with olive oil and season with salt and pepper.
3. Toss the beets until evenly coated with oil, salt, and pepper.
4. Roast in the preheated oven for about 45-50 minutes, or until the beets are tender when pierced with a fork. Stir halfway through cooking to ensure even roasting.
5. Once the beets are roasted, let them cool slightly.
6. In a large bowl, put together the roasted beets, baby spinach leaves, and toasted walnuts.
7. Gently toss the salad ingredients together.
8. Sprinkle crumbled feta cheese over the salad.
9. Drizzle with a little more olive oil if desired.
10. Season with additional salt and pepper to taste.
11. Serve the salad immediately while warm or at room temperature.

Nutritional Information:

- **Total Calories:** 250 kcal
- **Protein:** 8g
- **Carbohydrates:** 20g
- **Total Fat:** 15g
- **Fiber:** 6g
- **Sodium:** 200mg

Soft Mango Smoothie Bowl

Prep Time: 10 minutes | **Cook Time:** 0 minutes | **Servings:** 2

Ingredients:

- 1 ripe mango, peeled and diced
- 1/2 cup plain Greek yogurt
- 1/2 cup unsweetened almond milk
- 1 tablespoon chia seeds
- 1 tablespoon ground flaxseed
- 1 tablespoon honey (optional, omit for lower sugar content)
- Fresh berries and sliced almonds, for topping

Instructions:

1. Peel and dice the ripe mango.
2. In a blender, put together the diced mango, plain Greek yogurt, unsweetened almond milk, chia seeds, and ground flaxseed.
3. Blend until smooth and creamy. Adjust the consistency by adding more almond milk if needed.
4. Pour the smoothie into bowls.
5. Top each bowl with fresh berries and sliced almonds.
6. Serve the soft mango smoothie bowl immediately.

Nutritional Information:

- **Total Calories:** 180 kcal
- **Protein:** 8g
- **Carbohydrates:** 25g
- **Total Fat:** 5g
- **Fiber:** 6g
- **Sodium:** 50mg

Soft Cooked Polenta

Prep Time: 5 minutes | **Cook Time:** 30 minutes | **Servings:** 4

Ingredients:

- 1 cup polenta (cornmeal)
- 4 cups water or low-sodium vegetable broth
- Salt, to taste
- 1 tablespoon olive oil (optional for healthy fats)

Instructions:

1. In a bowl, put together the polenta with enough water to cover it by about 2 inches. Let it soak for at least 30 minutes to soften the grains.
2. In a medium saucepan, bring 4 cups of water or low-sodium vegetable broth to a boil.
3. Gradually whisk in the soaked polenta, stirring continuously to prevent clumps from forming.
4. Reduce the heat to low and simmer gently, stirring frequently with a wooden spoon, for about 30 minutes or until the polenta is thick and creamy. Add more water or broth if needed to achieve desired consistency.
5. Season with salt to taste. Stir in olive oil if using, for added healthy fats.
6. Serve the soft cooked polenta warm.

Nutritional Information:

- **Total Calories:** 150 kcal
- **Protein:** 3g
- **Carbohydrates:** 32g
- **Total Fat:** 2g
- **Fiber:** 2g
- **Sodium:** 5mg

Soft Steamed Carrots

Prep Time: 5 minutes | **Cook Time:** 10 minutes | **Servings:** 4

Ingredients:

- 4 large carrots, peeled and sliced into thick rounds

Instructions:

1. Peel the carrots and slice them into thick rounds.
2. Place the sliced carrots in a steamer basket over boiling water. Cover with a lid.
3. Steam the carrots for about 8-10 minutes, or until they are tender when pierced with a fork. Ensure they are soft enough for consumption in the soft food phase.
4. Take out the steamed carrots from the steamer basket and transfer them to a bowl. They should be soft and easy to mash with a fork.
5. Serve the soft steamed carrots warm as a side dish or as part of a soft food meal.

Nutritional Information:

- **Total Calories:** 50 kcal
- **Protein:** 1g
- **Carbohydrates:** 12g
- **Total Fat:** 0.3g
- **Fiber:** 3g
- **Sodium:** 40mg

Soft Cauliflower Mash

Prep Time: 10 minutes | **Cook Time:** 15 minutes | **Servings:** 4

Ingredients:

- 1 medium head of cauliflower, cut into florets
- 1/4 cup low-sodium vegetable broth
- 1/4 cup unsweetened almond milk
- Salt and pepper, to taste
- 1 tablespoon olive oil (optional for healthy fats)

Instructions:

1. Cut the cauliflower into florets, ensuring they are of similar size for even cooking.
2. Place the cauliflower florets in a steamer basket over boiling water. Cover with a lid.
3. Steam the cauliflower for about 10-12 minutes, or until very tender when pierced with a fork. They should be soft for mashing.
4. Transfer the steamed cauliflower to a large bowl. Add the low-sodium vegetable broth and unsweetened almond milk.
5. Use a potato masher or fork to mash the cauliflower until smooth and creamy. Add more vegetable broth or almond milk if needed to achieve desired consistency.
6. Season the cauliflower mash with salt and pepper to taste. Drizzle with olive oil if desired for healthy fats.
7. Serve the soft cauliflower mash warm as a side dish or as part of a soft food meal.

Nutritional Information:

- **Total Calories:** 60 kcal
- **Protein:** 3g
- **Carbohydrates:** 8g
- **Total Fat:** 2g
- **Fiber:** 4g
- **Sodium:** 50mg

Soft Black Bean Salad

Prep Time: 15 minutes | **Cook Time:** 0 minutes | **Servings:** 4

Ingredients:

- 1 can (15 oz) black beans, drained and rinsed
- 1 avocado, diced
- 1/2 red bell pepper, diced
- 1/2 cup cucumber, diced
- 1/4 cup red onion, finely chopped
- 1/4 cup fresh cilantro, chopped
- 1 tablespoon olive oil
- 1 tablespoon lime juice
- Salt and pepper, to taste

Instructions:

1. Drain and rinse the black beans thoroughly under cold water. Dice the avocado, red bell pepper, cucumber, and finely chop the red onion and cilantro.
2. In a large mixing bowl, put together the black beans, diced avocado, red bell pepper, cucumber, red onion, and cilantro.
3. Drizzle olive oil and lime juice over the salad ingredients.
4. Gently toss the salad until all ingredients are evenly coated with the dressing. Season with salt and pepper to taste.
5. Ensure all ingredients are diced finely to achieve a softer texture suitable for a soft food diet phase.
6. Serve the soft black bean salad immediately or refrigerate for later. Enjoy as a nutritious side dish or light meal.

Nutritional Information:

- **Total Calories:** 180 kcal
- **Protein:** 6g
- **Carbohydrates:** 19g
- **Total Fat:** 10g
- **Fiber:** 7g
- **Sodium:** 150mg

Soft Spinach Frittata

Prep Time: 15 minutes | **Cook Time:** 20 minutes | **Servings:** 4

Ingredients:

- 6 large eggs
- 1 cup fresh spinach leaves, chopped
- 1/2 cup low-fat cottage cheese
- 1/4 cup grated Parmesan cheese
- 1/4 cup onion, finely chopped
- 1 garlic clove, minced
- 1 tablespoon olive oil
- Salt and pepper, to taste

Instructions:

1. Chop the fresh spinach leaves, finely chop the onion, and mince the garlic clove.
2. In a non-stick skillet, heat olive oil over medium heat. Add chopped onion and minced garlic. Sauté until onion is translucent and fragrant, about 3-4 minutes.
3. Add chopped spinach to the skillet. Cook until spinach is wilted, about 2-3 minutes. Remove from heat and set aside.
4. In a mixing bowl, whisk together eggs, cottage cheese, and grated Parmesan cheese until well combined. Season with salt and pepper.
5. Pour the egg mixture over the sauteed spinach mixture in the skillet. Gently stir to evenly distribute the ingredients.
6. Return the skillet to low heat. Cook the frittata gently, without stirring, until the edges are set, about 8-10 minutes.
7. Ensure the frittata is cooked until set but still soft and moist inside, suitable for a soft food diet phase.
8. Once the frittata is cooked through, remove from heat. Allow it to cool slightly before slicing into wedges.
9. Serve the soft spinach frittata warm as a nutritious breakfast, lunch, or dinner option.

Nutritional Information:

- **Total Calories:** 170 kcal
- **Protein:** 15g
- **Carbohydrates:** 4g
- **Total Fat:** 10g
- **Fiber:** 1g
- **Sodium:** 260mg

Chapter 6: Solid Foods Phase

Grilled Chicken Breast

Prep Time: 10 minutes | **Cook Time:** 15 minutes | **Servings:** 4

Ingredients:

- 4 boneless, skinless chicken breasts
- 2 cloves garlic, minced
- 1 teaspoon dried oregano
- 1 teaspoon dried thyme
- 1/2 teaspoon paprika
- Salt and pepper, to taste
- 1 tablespoon olive oil

Instructions:

1. Preheat grill to medium-high heat.
2. In a small bowl, combine minced garlic, oregano, thyme, paprika, salt, and pepper.
3. Rub each chicken breast with the olive oil.
4. Sprinkle the seasoning mixture evenly over both sides of the chicken breasts.
5. Place seasoned chicken breasts on the preheated grill.
6. Grill for about 6-7 minutes on each side, or until the internal temperature reaches 165°F (75°C) and the juices run clear.
7. Remove chicken from grill and let it rest for a few minutes before serving.
8. Serve hot, optionally garnished with fresh herbs or a squeeze of lemon.

Nutritional Information:

- **Total Calories:** Approximately 180 calories per serving
- **Protein:** 30g
- **Carbohydrates:** 2g
- **Total Fat:** 5g
- **Fiber:** 0.5g
- **Sodium:** 80mg

Baked Salmon with Lemon

Prep Time: 10 minutes | **Cook Time:** 15 minutes | **Servings:** 4

Ingredients:

- 4 salmon fillets (about 4-6 ounces each), skinless
- 2 tablespoons olive oil
- 2 cloves garlic, minced
- 1 teaspoon dried dill
- 1/2 teaspoon paprika
- Salt and pepper, to taste
- 1 lemon, thinly sliced
- Fresh dill or parsley, for garnish

Instructions:

1. Preheat oven to 400°F (200°C).
2. Place salmon fillets on a baking sheet lined with parchment paper or lightly greased.
3. In a small bowl, mix together olive oil, minced garlic, dried dill, paprika, salt, and pepper.
4. Brush or spoon the olive oil mixture evenly over each salmon fillet.
5. Place a couple of lemon slices on each salmon fillet.
6. Bake in the preheated oven for 12-15 minutes, or until the salmon flakes easily with a fork and reaches an internal temperature of 145°F (63°C).
7. Remove from oven and let rest for a few minutes.
8. Garnish with fresh dill or parsley if desired.
9. Serve hot.

Nutritional Information:

- **Total Calories:** Approximately 250 calories per serving
- **Protein:** 30g
- **Carbohydrates:** 2g
- **Total Fat:** 13g
- **Fiber:** 0.5g
- **Sodium:** 70mg

Roasted Turkey Breast

Prep Time: 10 minutes | **Cook Time:** 1 hour 30 minutes | **Servings:** 6

Ingredients:

- 1 bone-in turkey breast (about 3 pounds)
- 2 tablespoons olive oil
- 2 cloves garlic, minced
- 1 teaspoon dried thyme
- 1 teaspoon dried rosemary
- 1 teaspoon dried sage
- Salt and pepper, to taste
- 1 lemon, sliced
- 1 onion, sliced
- 1 cup low-sodium chicken broth

Instructions:

1. Preheat oven to 350°F (175°C).
2. Place the turkey breast on a roasting pan or baking dish.
3. In a small bowl, combine olive oil, minced garlic, dried thyme, dried rosemary, dried sage, salt, and pepper.
4. Rub the olive oil mixture evenly over the turkey breast.
5. Arrange lemon slices and onion slices around the turkey breast.
6. Pour the chicken broth into the bottom of the roasting pan.
7. Cover the turkey breast loosely with aluminum foil.
8. Roast in the preheated oven for about 1 hour 30 minutes, or until the internal temperature of the thickest part of the breast reaches 165°F (75°C).
9. Remove from oven and let the turkey breast rest for 10-15 minutes before slicing.
10. Slice and serve warm, optionally with pan juices spooned over.

Nutritional Information:

- **Total Calories:** Approximately 220 calories per serving
- **Protein:** 30g
- **Carbohydrates:** 2g
- **Total Fat:** 10g
- **Fiber:** 0.5g
- **Sodium:** 90mg

Stuffed Bell Peppers

Prep Time: 20 minutes | **Cook Time:** 45 minutes | **Servings:** 4

Ingredients:

- 4 large bell peppers (any color), tops cut off and seeds removed
- 1/2 pound lean ground turkey
- 1/2 cup quinoa, rinsed
- 1 cup low-sodium chicken broth
- 1/2 onion, finely chopped
- 2 cloves garlic, minced
- 1 teaspoon olive oil
- 1 teaspoon dried oregano
- 1 teaspoon dried basil
- Salt and pepper, to taste
- 1/2 cup diced tomatoes (fresh or canned)
- 1/4 cup shredded low-fat mozzarella cheese (optional)

Instructions:

1. Preheat oven to 375°F (190°C).
2. Place the hollowed-out bell peppers upright in a baking dish.
3. In a small saucepan, bring the chicken broth to a boil.
4. Add quinoa, reduce heat to low, cover, and simmer for about 15 minutes until liquid is absorbed and quinoa is cooked.
5. In a skillet, heat olive oil over medium heat.
6. Add chopped onion and garlic, sauté until softened.
7. Add ground turkey, dried oregano, dried basil, salt, and pepper. Cook until turkey is browned and cooked through.
8. Stir in cooked quinoa and diced tomatoes into the turkey mixture. Mix adequately.
9. Spoon the turkey-quinoa mixture evenly into the hollowed-out bell peppers.
10. Cover the baking dish with foil and bake in the preheated oven for 30-35 minutes, or until the peppers are tender.
11. If desired, uncover the peppers in the last 10 minutes of baking and sprinkle shredded mozzarella cheese on top. Bake uncovered until cheese is melted and bubbly.
12. Remove from oven and let cool slightly before serving.

Nutritional Information:

- **Total Calories:** Approximately 250 calories per serving
- **Protein:** 22g
- **Carbohydrates:** 25g
- **Total Fat:** 7g
- **Fiber:** 5g
- **Sodium:** 150mg

Chicken and Vegetable Stir-Fry

Prep Time: 15 minutes | **Cook Time:** 15 minutes | **Servings:** 4

Ingredients:

- 1 pound boneless, skinless chicken breasts, thinly sliced
- 1 tablespoon olive oil
- 2 cloves garlic, minced
- 1 teaspoon grated fresh ginger
- 1 medium bell pepper, thinly sliced
- 1 medium zucchini, thinly sliced
- 1 cup broccoli florets
- 1 cup snap peas
- 2 tablespoons low-sodium soy sauce
- 1 tablespoon rice vinegar
- 1 teaspoon honey (optional, omit for lower sugar)
- Salt and pepper, to taste
- Fresh cilantro or green onions, for garnish

Instructions:

1. Heat olive oil in a large skillet or wok over medium-high heat.
2. Add minced garlic and grated ginger, sauté for 1 minute until fragrant.
3. Add sliced chicken breast to the skillet.
4. Stir-fry until chicken is cooked through and no longer pink, about 5-6 minutes.
5. Remove chicken from skillet and set aside.
6. In the same skillet, add bell pepper, zucchini, broccoli florets, and snap peas.
7. Stir-fry for 4-5 minutes until vegetables are crisp-tender.
8. Return cooked chicken to the skillet with the vegetables.
9. In a small bowl, mix together low-sodium soy sauce, rice vinegar, and honey (if using).
10. Pour the sauce over the chicken and vegetables. Stir adequately to combine and coat evenly.
11. Season with salt and pepper to taste.
12. Cook for an additional 1-2 minutes until everything is heated through.
13. Remove from heat and garnish with fresh cilantro or green onions.
14. Serve the stir-fry hot, optionally over brown rice or cauliflower rice.

Nutritional Information:

- **Total Calories:** Approximately 250 calories per serving
- **Protein:** 30g
- **Carbohydrates:** 12g
- **Total Fat:** 9g
- **Fiber:** 4g
- **Sodium:** 300mg

Baked Cod with Herbs

Prep Time: 10 minutes | **Cook Time:** 15 minutes | **Servings:** 4

Ingredients:

- 4 cod fillets (about 4-6 ounces each)
- 2 tablespoons olive oil
- 2 cloves garlic, minced
- 1 tablespoon fresh lemon juice
- 1 teaspoon dried thyme
- 1 teaspoon dried parsley
- Salt and pepper, to taste
- Lemon wedges, for serving
- Fresh parsley, chopped, for garnish

Instructions:

1. Preheat oven to 400°F (200°C).
2. Place the cod fillets in a single layer on a baking sheet lined with parchment paper or lightly greased.
3. In a small bowl, combine olive oil, minced garlic, lemon juice, dried thyme, dried parsley, salt, and pepper.
4. Brush or spoon the herb mixture evenly over each cod fillet.
5. Bake in the preheated oven for 12-15 minutes, or until the cod is opaque and flakes easily with a fork.
6. Remove from oven and let the cod rest for a few minutes.
7. Serve hot, garnished with lemon wedges and chopped fresh parsley.

Nutritional Information:

- **Total Calories:** Approximately 180 calories per serving
- **Protein:** 30g
- **Carbohydrates:** 1g
- **Total Fat:** 6g
- **Fiber:** 0g
- **Sodium:** 70mg

Turkey Meatballs

Prep Time: 15 minutes | **Cook Time:** 20 minutes | **Servings:** 4

Ingredients:

- 1 pound lean ground turkey
- 1/4 cup rolled oats, finely ground (use a food processor)
- 1/4 cup grated zucchini
- 1/4 cup finely chopped onion
- 1 clove garlic, minced
- 1/2 teaspoon dried oregano
- 1/2 teaspoon dried basil
- Salt and pepper, to taste
- 1 tablespoon olive oil
- 1 cup low-sodium chicken broth (for cooking)

Instructions:

1. In a large mixing bowl, combine ground turkey, finely ground rolled oats, grated zucchini, chopped onion, minced garlic, dried oregano, dried basil, salt, and pepper. Mix adequately until thoroughly combined.
2. Shape the mixture into small meatballs, about 1 inch in diameter.
3. In a large skillet, heat olive oil over medium heat.
4. Add the meatballs to the skillet in a single layer, ensuring they are not crowded.
5. Brown the meatballs on all sides, turning occasionally, for about 5 minutes.
6. Pour the low-sodium chicken broth into the skillet.
7. Reduce heat to low, cover, and simmer for 12-15 minutes, or until the meatballs are cooked through and reach an internal temperature of 165°F (75°C).
8. Remove from heat and let the meatballs rest for a few minutes before serving.
9. Serve hot as is or with a side of steamed vegetables.

Nutritional Information:

- **Total Calories:** Approximately 220 calories per serving
- **Protein:** 25g
- **Carbohydrates:** 6g
- **Total Fat:** 10g
- **Fiber:** 1g
- **Sodium:** 120mg

Quinoa and Veggie Salad

Prep Time: 15 minutes | **Cook Time:** 15 minutes | **Servings:** 4

Ingredients:

- 1 cup quinoa, rinsed
- 2 cups water or low-sodium vegetable broth
- 1 cup cherry tomatoes, halved
- 1 cucumber, diced
- 1 bell pepper (any color), diced
- 1/4 cup red onion, finely chopped
- 1/4 cup fresh parsley, chopped
- 2 tablespoons olive oil
- 2 tablespoons fresh lemon juice
- 1 teaspoon Dijon mustard
- Salt and pepper, to taste

Instructions:

1. In a medium saucepan, bring water or vegetable broth to a boil.
2. Add quinoa, reduce heat to low, cover, and simmer for about 12-15 minutes until liquid is absorbed and quinoa is tender.
3. Remove from heat and let cool.
4. In a large mixing bowl, combine cherry tomatoes, diced cucumber, diced bell pepper, red onion, and chopped parsley.
5. Add cooled quinoa to the bowl with vegetables.
6. In a small bowl, whisk together olive oil, lemon juice, Dijon mustard, salt, and pepper.
7. Pour the dressing over the quinoa and vegetables.
8. Toss gently until everything is well combined and evenly coated.
9. Cover the salad and refrigerate for at least 30 minutes to allow flavors to meld.
10. Serve chilled, optionally garnished with additional parsley.

Nutritional Information:

- **Total Calories:** Approximately 200 calories per serving
- **Protein:** 6g
- **Carbohydrates:** 30g
- **Total Fat:** 7g
- **Fiber:** 5g
- **Sodium:** 80mg

Grilled Shrimp Skewers

Prep Time: 20 minutes | **Cook Time:** 6 minutes | **Servings:** 4

Ingredients:

- 1 pound large shrimp, peeled and deveined
- 1 tablespoon olive oil
- 1 teaspoon smoked paprika
- 1/2 teaspoon garlic powder
- 1/2 teaspoon onion powder
- 1/2 teaspoon dried oregano
- 1/2 teaspoon dried thyme
- Salt and pepper, to taste
- Wooden or metal skewers

Instructions:

1. If using wooden skewers, soak them in water for 20-30 minutes to prevent burning.
2. Pat dry the peeled and deveined shrimp with paper towels.
3. In a bowl, combine olive oil, smoked paprika, garlic powder, onion powder, dried oregano, dried thyme, salt, and pepper.
4. Add shrimp to the bowl and toss to coat evenly with the seasoning mixture.
5. Thread the seasoned shrimp onto skewers, distributing evenly.
6. Preheat grill to medium-high heat.
7. Place the shrimp skewers on the grill and cook for about 2-3 minutes per side, or until shrimp are opaque and cooked through.
8. Remove shrimp skewers from the grill and let rest for a few minutes before serving.

Nutritional Information:

- **Total Calories:** Approximately 150 calories per serving
- **Protein:** 25g
- **Carbohydrates:** 1g
- **Total Fat:** 5g
- **Fiber:** 0g
- **Sodium:** 200mg

Baked Tofu with Soy Sauce

Prep Time: 10 minutes | **Cook Time:** 25 minutes | **Servings:** 4

Ingredients:

- 1 block (about 14 ounces) firm tofu, drained and pressed
- 2 tablespoons low-sodium soy sauce
- 1 tablespoon olive oil
- 1 clove garlic, minced
- 1 teaspoon grated fresh ginger
- 1/2 teaspoon sesame seeds
- Fresh cilantro or green onions, for garnish

Instructions:

1. Preheat the oven to 400°F (200°C).
2. Cut the pressed tofu into 1/2-inch-thick slices or cubes.
3. In a shallow dish, combine low-sodium soy sauce, olive oil, minced garlic, and grated fresh ginger.
4. Place tofu slices or cubes in the marinade, turning to coat evenly. Let marinate for 10 minutes.
5. Arrange marinated tofu in a single layer on a baking sheet lined with parchment paper or lightly greased.
6. Sprinkle sesame seeds evenly over the tofu.
7. Bake in the preheated oven for 20-25 minutes, flipping halfway through, until tofu is golden brown and slightly crisp.
8. Remove from the oven and let the baked tofu cool for a few minutes.
9. Garnish with fresh cilantro or green onions before serving.

Nutritional Information:

- **Total Calories:** Approximately 150 calories per serving
- **Protein:** 12g
- **Carbohydrates:** 5g
- **Total Fat:** 9g
- **Fiber:** 1g
- **Sodium:** 150mg

Stuffed Zucchini Boats

Prep Time: 20 minutes | **Cook Time:** 30 minutes | **Servings:** 4

Ingredients:

- 2 large zucchini
- 1/2 cup quinoa, cooked
- 1/2 cup cooked lean ground turkey
- 1/4 cup onion, finely chopped
- 1/4 cup bell pepper (any color), finely chopped
- 1 clove garlic, minced
- 1/2 teaspoon dried oregano
- 1/2 teaspoon dried basil
- Salt and pepper, to taste
- 1/4 cup shredded mozzarella cheese (optional)

Instructions:

1. Preheat oven to 400°F (200°C).
2. Cut each zucchini in half lengthwise. Scoop out the insides using a spoon, leaving about 1/4-inch thick shell. Chop the scooped zucchini flesh and set aside.
3. In a skillet, heat olive oil over medium heat. Add chopped onion, bell pepper, and minced garlic. Cook until softened, about 3-4 minutes.
4. Cook quinoa according to package instructions, if not already cooked.
5. Add chopped zucchini flesh, cooked quinoa, cooked lean ground turkey, dried oregano, dried basil, salt, and pepper to the skillet. Stir adequately to combine and cook for an additional 2-3 minutes until heated through.
6. Spoon the filling mixture evenly into the hollowed-out zucchini halves.
7. Place stuffed zucchini boats on a baking sheet lined with parchment paper or lightly greased.
8. If using cheese, sprinkle shredded mozzarella over the stuffed zucchini boats.
9. Bake in the preheated oven for 20-25 minutes, or until zucchini is tender and filling is heated through.
10. Remove from oven and let cool slightly before serving.

Nutritional Information:

- **Total Calories:** Approximately 180 calories per serving
- **Protein:** 15g
- **Carbohydrates:** 20g
- **Total Fat:** 5g
- **Fiber:** 4g
- **Sodium:** 80mg

Baked Chicken Parmesan

Prep Time: 20 minutes | **Cook Time:** 25 minutes | **Servings:** 4

Ingredients:

- 4 boneless, skinless chicken breasts
- 1/2 cup whole wheat breadcrumbs
- 1/4 cup grated Parmesan cheese
- 1 teaspoon dried oregano
- 1 teaspoon dried basil
- 1/2 teaspoon garlic powder
- 1/2 teaspoon onion powder
- Salt and pepper, to taste
- 1/2 cup marinara sauce (no added sugars)
- 1/2 cup shredded part-skim mozzarella cheese
- Fresh basil leaves, chopped, for garnish (optional)

Instructions:

1. Preheat oven to 400°F (200°C).
2. Place chicken breasts between two sheets of plastic wrap and gently pound to an even thickness using a meat mallet or rolling pin.
3. In a shallow dish, combine whole wheat breadcrumbs, grated Parmesan cheese, dried oregano, dried basil, garlic powder, onion powder, salt, and pepper.
4. Coat each chicken breast evenly with the breadcrumb mixture, pressing gently to adhere.
5. Place coated chicken breasts on a baking sheet lined with parchment paper or lightly greased.
6. Bake in the preheated oven for 20 minutes.
7. Remove chicken from the oven and top each breast with marinara sauce, spreading evenly.
8. Sprinkle shredded mozzarella cheese over the top of each chicken breast.
9. Return to the oven and bake for an additional 5 minutes, or until cheese is melted and bubbly.
10. Remove from oven and let chicken rest for a few minutes before serving.
11. Garnish with chopped fresh basil leaves, if desired.

Nutritional Information:

- **Total Calories:** Approximately 300 calories per serving
- **Protein:** 35g
- **Carbohydrates:** 10g
- **Total Fat:** 12g
- **Fiber:** 2g
- **Sodium:** 350mg

Grilled Vegetable Skewers

Prep Time: 20 minutes | **Cook Time:** 10 minutes | **Servings:** 4

Ingredients:

- 2 small zucchini, sliced into rounds
- 1 red bell pepper, cut into chunks
- 1 yellow bell pepper, cut into chunks
- 1 red onion, cut into chunks
- 8 cherry tomatoes
- 8 button mushrooms, halved
- 2 tablespoons olive oil
- 1 teaspoon dried oregano
- 1 teaspoon dried thyme
- Salt and pepper, to taste

Instructions:

1. If using wooden skewers, soak them in water for at least 30 minutes to prevent burning.
2. Preheat the grill to medium-high heat.
3. In a large bowl, combine zucchini, red bell pepper, yellow bell pepper, red onion, cherry tomatoes, and mushrooms.
4. Drizzle olive oil over the vegetables and sprinkle with dried oregano, dried thyme, salt, and pepper. Toss well to coat evenly.
5. Thread the marinated vegetables onto skewers, alternating between different vegetables for variety.
6. Place skewers on the preheated grill. Grill for about 5 minutes on each side, or until vegetables are tender and lightly charred.
7. Remove from the grill and let the skewers cool slightly before serving.

Nutritional Information:

- **Total Calories:** Approximately 120 calories per serving
- **Protein:** 3g
- **Carbohydrates:** 10g
- **Total Fat:** 8g
- **Fiber:** 3g
- **Sodium:** 15mg

Beef and Vegetable Stew

Prep Time: 20 minutes | **Cook Time:** 1 hour 30 minutes | **Servings:** 6

Ingredients:

- 1 pound lean beef stew meat, cut into cubes
- 2 tablespoons olive oil
- 1 onion, diced
- 2 cloves garlic, minced
- 2 carrots, peeled and sliced
- 2 celery stalks, sliced
- 1 red bell pepper, diced
- 1 zucchini, diced
- 1 cup green beans, trimmed and cut into 1-inch pieces
- 1 teaspoon dried thyme
- 1 teaspoon dried rosemary
- 1 bay leaf
- 4 cups low-sodium beef broth
- Salt and pepper, to taste

Instructions:

1. In a large pot or Dutch oven, heat olive oil over medium-high heat.
2. Add beef cubes and cook until browned on all sides. Remove beef from pot and set aside.
3. In the same pot, add diced onion and minced garlic. Sauté for 2-3 minutes until softened.
4. Add carrots, celery, red bell pepper, zucchini, and green beans. Cook for an additional 5 minutes, stirring occasionally.
5. Return the browned beef cubes to the pot.
6. Add dried thyme, dried rosemary, bay leaf, and low-sodium beef broth. Season with salt and pepper to taste.
7. Bring the stew to a boil, then reduce heat to low. Cover and simmer for 1 hour, stirring occasionally, until beef is tender and flavors are melded.
8. Remove bay leaf before serving.
9. Serve hot, adjusting seasoning if necessary.

Nutritional Information:

- **Total Calories:** Approximately 250 calories per serving
- **Protein:** 25g
- **Carbohydrates:** 15g
- **Total Fat:** 9g
- **Fiber:** 4g
- **Sodium:** 150mg

Chicken Fajita Bowl

Prep Time: 15 minutes | **Cook Time:** 20 minutes | **Servings:** 4

Ingredients:

- 1 pound boneless, skinless chicken breasts, thinly sliced
- 1 tablespoon olive oil
- 1 onion, thinly sliced
- 1 red bell pepper, thinly sliced
- 1 green bell pepper, thinly sliced
- 1 yellow bell pepper, thinly sliced
- 1 tablespoon chili powder
- 1 teaspoon ground cumin
- 1 teaspoon smoked paprika
- Salt and pepper, to taste
- 1 cup cooked quinoa
- 1 cup black beans, drained and rinsed
- 1 avocado, sliced
- Fresh cilantro, for garnish
- Lime wedges, for serving

Instructions:

1. Heat olive oil in a large skillet over medium-high heat.
2. Add sliced chicken breasts and cook until browned and cooked through, about 5-7 minutes. Remove chicken from skillet and set aside.
3. In the same skillet, add sliced onion and bell peppers. Cook until softened and slightly caramelized, about 5-7 minutes.
4. Return the cooked chicken to the skillet with the vegetables.
5. Sprinkle chili powder, ground cumin, smoked paprika, salt, and pepper over the chicken and vegetables. Stir adequately to combine and cook for an additional 2-3 minutes until everything is heated through and well coated with seasonings.
6. Divide cooked quinoa evenly among serving bowls.
7. Top each bowl with the chicken and vegetable mixture.
8. Add black beans and avocado slices to each bowl.
9. Garnish with fresh cilantro and serve with lime wedges.
10. Serve hot, optionally squeezing lime juice over the bowls before eating.

Nutritional Information (per serving):

- **Total Calories:** Approximately 350 calories
- **Protein:** 30g
- **Carbohydrates:** 30g
- **Total Fat:** 12g
- **Fiber:** 10g
- **Sodium:** 200mg

Stuffed Portobello Mushrooms

Prep Time: 15 minutes | **Cook Time:** 20 minutes | **Servings:** 4

Ingredients:

- 4 large Portobello mushrooms
- 1 tablespoon olive oil
- 1 small onion, finely diced
- 2 cloves garlic, minced
- 1 red bell pepper, finely diced
- 1 zucchini, finely diced
- 1/2 cup cherry tomatoes, diced
- 1/2 cup quinoa, cooked
- 1/4 cup fresh parsley, chopped
- Salt and pepper, to taste
- 1/4 cup grated Parmesan cheese (optional)
- Fresh basil leaves, for garnish

Instructions:

1. Preheat oven to 375°F (190°C).
2. Clean the Portobello mushrooms and take out the stems. Use a spoon to gently scrape out the gills and create space for the stuffing.
3. Heat olive oil in a skillet over medium heat. Add onion and garlic, sauté until softened, about 3-4 minutes.
4. Add diced red bell pepper and zucchini, cook for an additional 3-4 minutes until vegetables are tender.
5. Stir in cherry tomatoes and cooked quinoa. Cook for 2 minutes until heated through.
6. Remove from heat and stir in chopped parsley. Season with salt and pepper to taste.
7. Place the Portobello mushrooms on a baking sheet lined with parchment paper.
8. Divide the vegetable quinoa mixture evenly among the mushrooms, filling the caps generously.
9. Optionally, sprinkle grated Parmesan cheese on top of each stuffed mushroom.
10. Bake in the preheated oven for 15-20 minutes, or until the mushrooms are tender and the filling is heated through.
11. Remove from the oven and garnish with fresh basil leaves.
12. Serve hot as a main dish.

Nutritional Information (per serving):

- **Total Calories:** Approximately 150 calories
- **Protein:** 7g
- **Carbohydrates:** 20g
- **Total Fat:** 4g
- **Fiber:** 4g
- **Sodium:** 80mg

Baked Eggplant Parmesan

Prep Time: 30 minutes | **Cook Time:** 40 minutes | **Servings:** 4

Ingredients:

- 1 large eggplant, sliced into 1/2-inch rounds
- 1 cup whole wheat breadcrumbs
- 1/2 cup grated Parmesan cheese
- 2 eggs
- 1 cup marinara sauce
- 1 cup part-skim mozzarella cheese, shredded
- Fresh basil leaves, for garnish
- Salt and pepper, to taste
- Olive oil cooking spray

Instructions:

1. Preheat the oven to 400°F (200°C). Line a baking sheet with parchment paper and lightly coat it with olive oil cooking spray.
2. Slice the eggplant into 1/2-inch rounds. Lay them on the prepared baking sheet and sprinkle both sides with salt. Let them sit for about 15 minutes to release excess moisture. Pat dry with paper towels.
3. In a shallow bowl, beat the eggs with a fork until well mixed. In another shallow bowl, put together the whole wheat breadcrumbs with grated Parmesan cheese.
4. Dip each eggplant slice into the beaten eggs, allowing any excess to drip off, then coat both sides with the breadcrumb mixture. Place the breaded slices back onto the baking sheet.
5. Lightly spray the tops of the breaded eggplant slices with olive oil cooking spray. Bake in the preheated oven for 20-25 minutes, flipping halfway through, until golden brown and crispy.
6. Reduce the oven temperature to 375°F (190°C). Spread 1/4 cup of marinara sauce evenly in the bottom of a baking dish.
7. Arrange half of the baked eggplant slices in a single layer over the sauce. Top each slice with a spoonful of marinara sauce and a sprinkle of shredded mozzarella cheese.
8. Repeat with another layer of eggplant, marinara sauce, and mozzarella cheese.
9. Cover the baking dish loosely with foil and bake in the oven for 15-20 minutes, until the cheese is melted and bubbly.
10. Remove from the oven and let it cool slightly before serving.
11. Garnish with fresh basil leaves and season with black pepper, if desired.

Nutritional Information (per serving):

- **Total Calories:** Approximately 280 calories
- **Protein:** 16g
- **Carbohydrates:** 30g
- **Total Fat:** 10g
- **Fiber:** 7g
- **Sodium:** 450mg

Turkey and Avocado Wrap

Prep Time: 15 minutes | **Cook Time:** 0 minutes | **Servings:** 2

Ingredients:

- 4 large lettuce leaves (such as romaine or butter lettuce)
- 8 ounces cooked turkey breast, sliced
- 1 avocado, sliced
- 1/2 cucumber, thinly sliced
- 1/2 red bell pepper, thinly sliced
- 1/4 cup shredded carrots
- 1/4 cup hummus
- 1 tablespoon Dijon mustard
- Salt and pepper, to taste

Instructions:

1. Lay out 2 large lettuce leaves per wrap on a clean surface.
2. Spread 2 tablespoons of hummus evenly over each lettuce leaf.
3. Layer the sliced turkey breast, avocado slices, cucumber slices, red bell pepper slices, and shredded carrots evenly over the hummus on each wrap.
4. Drizzle each wrap with 1/2 tablespoon of Dijon mustard.
5. Season with salt and pepper to taste.
6. Fold the sides of each lettuce leaf over the filling, then roll tightly from bottom to top to form a wrap.
7. Cut each wrap in half diagonally and serve immediately.

Nutritional Information (per serving):

- **Total Calories:** Approximately 250 calories
- **Protein:** 20g
- **Carbohydrates:** 15g
- **Total Fat:** 12g
- **Fiber:** 8g
- **Sodium:** 300mg

Chicken Caesar Salad

Prep Time: 20 minutes | **Cook Time:** 15 minutes | **Servings:** 2

Ingredients:

- 2 boneless, skinless chicken breasts
- 1 tablespoon olive oil
- Salt and pepper, to taste
- 1 head romaine lettuce, chopped
- 1/4 cup grated Parmesan cheese
- 1/4 cup Caesar salad dressing (preferably low-fat or homemade)
- 1/4 cup cherry tomatoes, halved
- 1/4 cup cucumber, diced
- 1/4 cup croutons (optional)

Instructions:

1. Preheat the oven to 400°F (200°C).
2. Rub the chicken breasts with olive oil and season with salt and pepper.
3. Place the chicken on a baking sheet and bake for 15-20 minutes, or until cooked through and no longer pink in the center. Alternatively, you can grill or pan-sear the chicken until fully cooked. Once done, let it rest for a few minutes before slicing.
4. In a large mixing bowl, put together the chopped romaine lettuce, grated Parmesan cheese, cherry tomatoes, and diced cucumber.
5. Slice the cooked chicken breasts into thin strips.
6. Add the sliced chicken to the salad bowl.
7. Drizzle the Caesar salad dressing over the salad ingredients.
8. Gently toss the salad until all ingredients are evenly coated with the dressing.
9. Divide the salad into two bowls or plates.
10. Optionally, sprinkle croutons over the top for added texture.
11. Enjoy your Chicken Caesar Salad immediately while it's fresh.

Nutritional Information (per serving):

- **Total Calories:** Approximately 350 calories
- **Protein:** 35g
- **Carbohydrates:** 10g
- **Total Fat:** 18g
- **Fiber:** 5g
- **Sodium:** 450mg

Baked Tilapia with Herbs

Prep Time: 10 minutes | **Cook Time:** 15 minutes | **Servings:** 2

Ingredients:

- 2 tilapia fillets (about 4-6 ounces each)
- 1 tablespoon olive oil
- 1 tablespoon fresh lemon juice
- 1 teaspoon fresh thyme leaves
- 1 teaspoon fresh rosemary leaves, chopped
- Salt and pepper, to taste
- 1 clove garlic, minced
- Lemon wedges, for serving

Instructions:

1. Preheat your oven to 400°F (200°C). Lightly grease a baking dish with olive oil or cooking spray.
2. Pat dry the tilapia fillets with paper towels to remove excess moisture.
3. Place the tilapia fillets in the prepared baking dish.
4. Drizzle olive oil and fresh lemon juice over the tilapia fillets.
5. Sprinkle with fresh thyme leaves, chopped rosemary, minced garlic, salt, and pepper.
6. Bake the tilapia in the preheated oven for about 12-15 minutes, or until the fish is opaque and easily flakes with a fork.
7. Take out the baked tilapia from the oven.
8. Serve hot with lemon wedges on the side for extra flavor.

Nutritional Information (per serving):

- **Total Calories:** Approximately 180 calories
- **Protein:** 25g
- **Carbohydrates:** 1g
- **Total Fat:** 8g
- **Fiber:** 0g
- **Sodium:** 80mg

Veggie and Hummus Wrap

Prep Time: 15 minutes | **Cook Time:** 0 minutes | **Servings:** 2

Ingredients:

- 2 whole wheat or low-carb tortilla wraps
- 1/2 cup hummus (preferably homemade or low sodium)
- 1 cup mixed vegetables (such as lettuce, spinach, bell peppers, cucumbers, tomatoes), thinly sliced or shredded
- 1/2 cup shredded carrots
- 1/4 cup sliced red onion
- Fresh herbs (optional), such as parsley or cilantro
- Salt and pepper, to taste

Instructions:

1. Lay out the tortilla wraps on a clean surface.
2. Spread 1/4 cup of hummus evenly over each tortilla wrap.
3. Evenly distribute the mixed vegetables, shredded carrots, sliced red onion, and fresh herbs over the hummus layer on each tortilla.
4. Season with salt and pepper to taste.
5. Roll up each tortilla tightly into a wrap.
6. Slice each wrap in half diagonally.
7. Serve the Veggie and Hummus Wraps immediately.

Nutritional Information (per serving):

- **Total Calories:** Approximately 250 calories
- **Protein:** 10g
- **Carbohydrates:** 30g
- **Total Fat:** 10g
- **Fiber:** 7g
- **Sodium:** 200mg

Grilled Pork Tenderloin

Prep Time: 10 minutes | **Cook Time:** 20 minutes | **Servings:** 4

Ingredients:

- 1 pound pork tenderloin
- 2 cloves garlic, minced
- 1 tsp dried thyme
- 1 tsp dried rosemary
- 1/2 tsp paprika
- Salt and pepper, to taste
- 1 tbsp olive oil

Instructions:

1. Preheat your grill to medium-high heat.
2. Trim any excess fat from the pork tenderloin.
3. In a small bowl, combine minced garlic, dried thyme, dried rosemary, paprika, salt, and pepper.
4. Rub the pork tenderloin all over with olive oil.
5. Sprinkle the seasoning mixture evenly over the pork, rubbing it into the meat.
6. Place the pork tenderloin on the preheated grill. Grill for about 18-20 minutes, turning occasionally, until the internal temperature reaches 145°F (63°C) for medium rare or up to 160°F (71°C) for medium, depending on your preference.
7. Take out the pork from the grill and let it rest for 5 minutes before slicing.
8. Slice the pork tenderloin into thin slices and serve immediately.

Nutritional Information (per serving):

- **Total Calories:** Approximately 200 calories
- **Protein:** 25g
- **Carbohydrates:** 1g
- **Total Fat:** 10g
- **Fiber:** 0g
- **Sodium:** 60mg

Beef and Broccoli Stir-Fry

Prep Time: 15 minutes | **Cook Time:** 15 minutes | **Servings:** 4

Ingredients:

- 1 pound beef sirloin, thinly sliced
- 2 cups broccoli florets
- 1 red bell pepper, thinly sliced
- 1 yellow bell pepper, thinly sliced
- 1 onion, thinly sliced
- 2 cloves garlic, minced
- 1-inch piece of ginger, minced
- 1/4 cup low-sodium soy sauce
- 2 tbsp oyster sauce
- 1 tbsp cornstarch
- 1 tbsp olive oil
- Salt and pepper, to taste

Instructions:

1. In a bowl, combine the beef slices with minced garlic, minced ginger, soy sauce, oyster sauce, cornstarch, salt, and pepper. Mix adequately and let it marinate for 10 minutes.
2. Heat olive oil in a large skillet or wok over medium-high heat. Add the sliced onion, red bell pepper, yellow bell pepper, and broccoli florets. Stir-fry for 5-6 minutes until the vegetables are tender-crisp. Take out the vegetables from the skillet and set aside.
3. In the same skillet or wok, add the marinated beef slices along with the marinade. Stir-fry for 4-5 minutes until the beef is cooked through and the sauce has thickened.
4. Add the cooked vegetables back into the skillet with the beef. Stir-fry for an additional 1-2 minutes until everything is heated through and well combined.
5. Taste and adjust seasoning with salt and pepper if needed.
6. Serve the Beef and Broccoli Stir-Fry hot over a bed of brown rice or quinoa, if desired.

Nutritional Information (per serving):

- **Total Calories:** Approximately 300 calories
- **Protein:** 25g
- **Carbohydrates:** 15g
- **Total Fat:** 15g
- **Fiber:** 4g
- **Sodium:** 400mg

Baked Chicken Thighs

Prep Time: 10 minutes | **Cook Time:** 35 minutes | **Servings:** 4

Ingredients:

- 4 boneless, skinless chicken thighs
- 2 tablespoons olive oil
- 1 teaspoon dried thyme
- 1 teaspoon dried rosemary
- 1 teaspoon garlic powder
- 1 teaspoon onion powder
- 1/2 teaspoon paprika
- Salt and pepper, to taste

Instructions:

1. Preheat your oven to 400°F (200°C). Line a baking sheet with parchment paper or lightly grease it with olive oil.
2. In a small bowl, mix together the dried thyme, dried rosemary, garlic powder, onion powder, paprika, salt, and pepper.
3. Rub the chicken thighs with olive oil and then evenly coat them with the seasoning mixture.
4. Place the seasoned chicken thighs on the prepared baking sheet. Bake in the preheated oven for 25-30 minutes, or until the internal temperature reaches 165°F (75°C) and the chicken is cooked through.
5. Take out the chicken thighs from the oven and let them rest for 5 minutes before serving.

Nutritional Information (per serving):

- **Total Calories:** Approximately 250 calories
- **Protein:** 25g
- **Carbohydrates:** 2g
- **Total Fat:** 15g
- **Fiber:** 1g
- **Sodium:** 200mg

Veggie and Quinoa Bowl

Prep Time: 15 minutes | **Cook Time:** 20 minutes | **Servings:** 4

Ingredients:

- 1 cup quinoa, rinsed
- 2 cups water
- 1 tablespoon olive oil
- 1 cup cherry tomatoes, halved
- 1 cucumber, diced
- 1 red bell pepper, diced
- 1 avocado, diced
- 1/4 cup red onion, finely chopped
- 1/4 cup fresh parsley, chopped
- 1 lemon, juiced
- 1 teaspoon dried oregano
- Salt and pepper, to taste

Instructions:

1. In a medium saucepan, bring the water to a boil. Add the rinsed quinoa, reduce the heat to low, cover, and simmer for about 15 minutes or until the water is absorbed and the quinoa is tender. Fluff with a fork and let it cool.
2. While the quinoa is cooking, prepare the vegetables. Halve the cherry tomatoes, dice the cucumber, red bell pepper, and avocado, finely chop the red onion, and chop the fresh parsley.
3. In a large mixing bowl, put together the cooked and cooled quinoa with the cherry tomatoes, cucumber, red bell pepper, avocado, red onion, and parsley.
4. In a small bowl, whisk together the olive oil, fresh lemon juice, dried oregano, salt, and pepper.
5. Pour the dressing over the quinoa and vegetable mixture. Toss gently to combine and coat evenly.
6. Divide the veggie and quinoa mixture into bowls and serve immediately.

Nutritional Information (per serving):

- **Total Calories:** Approximately 250 calories
- **Protein:** 7g
- **Carbohydrates:** 35g
- **Total Fat:** 10g
- **Fiber:** 8g
- **Sodium:** 50mg

Grilled Salmon Salad

Prep Time: 15 minutes | **Cook Time:** 10 minutes | **Servings:** 4

Ingredients:

- 4 salmon fillets (about 4 ounces each)
- 1 tablespoon olive oil
- 1 lemon, juiced
- 1 teaspoon dried dill
- Salt and pepper, to taste
- 8 cups mixed greens (such as spinach, arugula, and romaine)
- 1 cup cherry tomatoes, halved
- 1 cucumber, diced
- 1/4 red onion, thinly sliced
- 1 avocado, diced
- 1/4 cup fresh parsley, chopped
- 2 tablespoons olive oil (for dressing)
- 1 tablespoon balsamic vinegar
- Salt and pepper, to taste (for dressing)

Instructions:

1. Preheat the grill to medium-high heat.
2. Rub the salmon fillets with olive oil, lemon juice, dried dill, salt, and pepper.
3. Place the salmon on the grill and cook for about 4-5 minutes on each side, or until the salmon is opaque and flakes easily with a fork. Remove from the grill and let it cool slightly.
4. In a large bowl, put together the mixed greens, cherry tomatoes, diced cucumber, thinly sliced red onion, diced avocado, and chopped fresh parsley.
5. In a small bowl, whisk together the olive oil, balsamic vinegar, salt, and pepper.
6. Divide the salad mixture into four serving bowls.
7. Top each bowl with a grilled salmon fillet.
8. Drizzle the dressing evenly over the salads.
9. Serve immediately, optionally with an extra lemon wedge on the side.

Nutritional Information (per serving):

- **Total Calories:** Approximately 350 calories
- **Protein:** 30g
- **Carbohydrates:** 10g
- **Total Fat:** 20g
- **Fiber:** 6g
- **Sodium:** 150mg

Baked Falafel with Tzatziki

Prep Time: 20 minutes | **Cook Time:** 25 minutes | **Servings:** 4

Ingredients:

For the Falafel:

- 1 can (15 ounces) chickpeas, drained and rinsed
- 1 small onion, diced
- 2 cloves garlic, minced
- 1/4 cup fresh parsley, chopped
- 1/4 cup fresh cilantro, chopped
- 1 teaspoon ground cumin
- 1 teaspoon ground coriander
- 1/2 teaspoon baking powder
- 1 tablespoon olive oil
- Salt and pepper, to taste

For the Tzatziki:

- 1 cup plain Greek yogurt (non-fat or low-fat)
- 1/2 cucumber, grated and drained
- 1 clove garlic, minced
- 1 tablespoon fresh dill, chopped
- 1 tablespoon fresh lemon juice
- Salt and pepper, to taste

Instructions:

1. Preheat your oven to 375°F (190°C). Line a baking sheet with parchment paper or lightly grease it with olive oil.

2. In a food processor, put together the chickpeas, diced onion, minced garlic, fresh parsley, fresh cilantro, ground cumin, ground coriander, baking powder, olive oil, salt, and pepper. Pulse until the mixture is well combined but still slightly chunky. If the mixture is too wet, you can add a little bit of flour or breadcrumbs.

3. Scoop out about 2 tablespoons of the mixture and form it into small patties or balls. Place them on the prepared baking sheet.

4. Bake in the preheated oven for 20-25 minutes, flipping halfway through, until the falafel are golden brown and crispy on the outside.

5. While the falafel are baking, prepare the tzatziki sauce. In a medium bowl, put together the plain Greek yogurt, grated cucumber, minced garlic, fresh dill, fresh lemon juice, salt, and pepper. Mix adequately and refrigerate until ready to serve.

6. Serve the baked falafel warm with the prepared tzatziki sauce on the side. Optionally, serve with whole grain pita bread and a side salad.

Nutritional Information (per serving):

- **Total Calories:** Approximately 220 calories
- **Protein:** 12g
- **Carbohydrates:** 30g
- **Total Fat:** 7g
- **Fiber:** 8g
- **Sodium:** 250mg

Turkey and Veggie Skillet

Prep Time: 15 minutes | **Cook Time:** 20 minutes | **Servings:** 4

Ingredients:

- 1 pound ground turkey
- 1 tablespoon olive oil
- 1 onion, diced
- 2 cloves garlic, minced
- 1 red bell pepper, diced
- 1 zucchini, diced
- 1 cup broccoli florets
- 1 cup cherry tomatoes, halved
- 1 teaspoon dried oregano
- 1 teaspoon dried basil
- Salt and pepper, to taste
- Fresh parsley, chopped, for garnish

Instructions:

1. Heat olive oil in a large skillet over medium-high heat.
2. Add the ground turkey to the skillet. Cook until browned and fully cooked, breaking it apart with a spatula, about 5-7 minutes. Take out the turkey from the skillet and set aside.
3. In the same skillet, add the diced onion and minced garlic. Sauté until softened, about 2-3 minutes.
4. Add the diced red bell pepper, diced zucchini, and broccoli florets. Cook until the vegetables are tender, about 5-7 minutes.
5. Return the cooked turkey to the skillet with the vegetables.
6. Add the halved cherry tomatoes, dried oregano, and dried basil. Stir to combine and cook for an additional 2-3 minutes until everything is heated through.
7. Season with salt and pepper to taste.
8. Garnish with fresh chopped parsley.
9. Serve hot, optionally over a bed of brown rice or quinoa for added carbs and fiber.

Nutritional Information (per serving):

- **Total Calories:** Approximately 250 calories
- **Protein:** 25g
- **Carbohydrates:** 12g
- **Total Fat:** 12g
- **Fiber:** 4g
- **Sodium:** 75mg

Chapter 7: Bariatric Meal Preparation Tips

Grocery Shopping Tips for Bariatric Patients

Grocery shopping after surgery might feel different as you focus on buying nutrient-dense foods in smaller quantities. Here are some tips to make your shopping trips efficient and bariatric-friendly:

1. **Make a List**

   - Before heading to the store, create a detailed shopping list based on your meal plan for the week. This helps you stay focused and avoid impulse buys.

   - Organize your list by store sections (produce, dairy, protein, etc.) to streamline your shopping experience.

2. **Focus on Whole Foods**

   - Prioritize fresh, whole foods over processed and packaged items. Fill your cart with fresh fruits, vegetables, lean proteins, and whole grains.

   - Avoid products with added sugars, unhealthy fats, and artificial ingredients.

3. **Read Labels Carefully**

   - Check nutrition labels and ingredient lists. Look for items high in protein and low in added sugars and unhealthy fats.

   - Be cautious with products marketed as "low-fat" or "sugar-free," as they might contain other additives or have higher calorie counts.

4. **Shop the Perimeter**

   - The grocery store's perimeter typically houses fresh produce, dairy, and meats, while the aisles contain more processed foods.

   - Spend more time shopping the perimeter to pick the healthiest options.

5. **Buy in Bulk Wisely**

   - While buying in bulk can save money, consider your reduced food intake. Purchase items like frozen vegetables, lean meats, and pantry staples in bulk, but watch expiration dates.

6. **Stock Up on Essentials**

   - Keep your pantry stocked with essentials like low-sodium broths, canned beans, and whole grains. These items can be the foundation of many quick and healthy meals.

   - Invest in various herbs and spices to add flavor to your dishes without extra calories.

Time-Saving Meal Prep Techniques

Meal prep can be a lifesaver for staying on track with your diet, especially when you have a busy schedule. Here are some time-saving techniques to make meal prep efficient and effective:

1. **Batch Cooking**
   - Cook large batches of staple foods like grilled chicken, quinoa, or roasted vegetables that you can use in multiple meals throughout the week.
   - Divide batch-cooked items into single-serving portions and store them in the refrigerator or freezer for easy access.

2. **Prep Ingredients Ahead**
   - Wash, chop, and store vegetables and fruits immediately after you bring them home. This makes them readily available for snacks or quick meals.
   - Marinate proteins ahead of time so they are ready to cook when needed.

3. **Use Kitchen Gadgets**
   - Utilize time-saving kitchen gadgets like slow cookers, pressure cookers, and food processors to speed up meal prep.
   - Slow cookers can be set in the morning to have a meal ready by dinner, while pressure cookers can cook meals quickly, saving you valuable time.

4. **Organize Your Kitchen**
   - Keep your kitchen organized and stocked with essential tools and containers. A tidy, well-stocked kitchen makes meal prep more efficient and enjoyable.
   - Store prepped ingredients and meals in clear, labeled containers, which make it easy to find what you need.

5. **Plan for Convenience**
   - Prepare grab-and-go snacks like portioned-out nuts, yogurt cups, or fruit slices for busy days.
   - Cook and portion meals into individual containers that you can reheat for quick lunches or dinners.

6. **Stay Consistent**
   - Make meal prep a regular part of your routine. Set aside a specific time each week to prep meals, making it a non-negotiable part of your schedule.
   - Consistency in meal prepping will help establish healthy habits and ensure you always have nutritious options available.

By incorporating these meal planning and prep tips into your routine, you'll be well-equipped to navigate your post-surgery dietary journey. With thoughtful planning, smart shopping, and efficient meal prep, maintaining a healthy diet will become a seamless part of your new lifestyle.

Chapter 8: Tackling Common Challenges

Managing Food Intolerance

After gastric sleeve surgery, your digestive system undergoes quite a transformation. Some foods that you used to love might now cause discomfort. Identifying and managing food intolerances is vital to ensure a smooth recovery and maintain a healthy diet.

1. **Spot the Problem Foods**

    - Pay attention to how your body reacts to different foods. Keep a food diary to track what you eat and note any adverse reactions like bloating, nausea, or discomfort.

    - Common culprits include high-fat, high-sugar, and very fibrous foods. Spicy foods and carbonated beverages can also cause issues.

2. **Ease Into New Foods**

    - When reintroducing solid foods, do it slowly and one at a time. This will help you pinpoint any specific intolerances.

    - Start with small portions and gradually increase them as you assess your tolerance levels.

3. **Try Different Cooking Methods**

    - Some foods might be easier to tolerate if prepared differently. For instance, steaming vegetables instead of eating them raw can make them easier to digest.

    - Opt for baking, grilling, and steaming over frying to reduce fat content and enhance digestibility.

4. **Get Professional Help**

    - If you're having persistent issues with certain foods, consult a dietitian or your healthcare provider. They can provide personalized guidance and suggest alternatives.

    - Sometimes, food intolerances are temporary and may improve as your body adjusts to its new digestive dynamics.

5. **Stay Hydrated**

    - Drinking enough water is crucial, but avoid gulping large amounts during meals, as this can cause discomfort. Sip fluids throughout the day instead.

    - Choose non-carbonated, non-caffeinated, and low-sugar beverages to stay hydrated without upsetting your stomach.

Managing Emotional Eating

Emotional eating is a common challenge, especially after a major life change like gastric sleeve surgery. Learning to handle your emotions without turning to food is critical for long-term success.

1. **Identify Emotional Triggers**
   - Recognize the emotions and situations that lead to overeating. Common triggers include stress, boredom, sadness, and even celebrations.
   - Keeping a journal to document your feelings and eating patterns can help you identify and address these triggers.

2. **Find Healthy Coping Mechanisms**
   - Replace emotional eating with healthier strategies. This could include activities like walking, meditating, reading, or engaging in a hobby you enjoy.
   - Physical activity can be a great way to relieve stress and improve your mood without turning to food.

3. **Practice Mindful Eating**
   - Focus on eating mindfully by paying full attention to your meals and avoiding distractions like TV or phones while eating.
   - To prevent overeating, eat slowly, savor each bite, and listen to your body's hunger and fullness cues.

4. **Seek Support**
   - Surround yourself with supportive friends and family who understand your goals and can offer encouragement.
   - Consider joining a support group for bariatric patients. Sharing experiences and strategies with others in similar situations can be beneficial.

5. **Professional Help**
   - If emotional eating becomes a persistent issue, seek help from a mental health professional. They can provide valuable tools and strategies to cope with emotions healthily.
   - Therapies like cognitive-behavioral therapy (CBT) can be particularly effective in addressing emotional eating patterns.

Staying Hydrated and Active

Maintaining hydration and staying physically active are crucial components of a healthy lifestyle post-surgery. They play a significant role in your overall well-being and weight loss journey.

1. **Importance of Hydration**

- Drinking enough water is essential for digestion, nutrient absorption, and overall health. It helps prevent dehydration, which can cause fatigue, dizziness, and kidney issues.
- Aim to drink at least 64 ounces of water per day. Carry a water bottle with you to remind yourself to sip regularly.

2. **Tips for Staying Hydrated**

   - Drink small amounts frequently throughout the day rather than large quantities at once. This is easier on your new stomach size and helps prevent discomfort.
   - Infuse water with fruits, herbs, or cucumber slices for added flavor without extra calories. Herbal teas and broths are also good options for variety.

3. **Incorporate Physical Activity**

   - Regular physical activity helps you lose weight, improves your mood, and boosts overall health. Start with gentle exercises like walking or swimming and gradually increase the intensity as you build stamina.
   - Aim for at least 150 minutes of moderate-intensity exercise per week. Find activities you enjoy to make exercise a fun part of your routine.

4. **Exercise Tips Post-Surgery**

   - Begin with low-impact activities and listen to your body. Avoid high-intensity or strenuous exercises until your doctor clears you for such activities.
   - Incorporate strength training exercises to build muscle mass, which can help boost metabolism and support weight loss.

5. **Stay Motivated**

   - Set realistic and achievable fitness goals. Celebrate milestones, no matter how small, to keep yourself motivated.
   - Consider working with a fitness professional who has experience with bariatric patients. They can provide a tailored exercise plan that suits your needs and abilities.

By addressing common challenges such as food intolerance, emotional eating, and the need for hydration and physical activity, you'll be better equipped to navigate your post-surgery journey.

Conclusion

Congratulations on making the critical decision to improve your health and well-being with gastric sleeve surgery. *"The Easy Gastric Sleeve Bariatric Cookbook"* has been carefully designed to assist you on your transformative journey, equipping you with the necessary knowledge, tools, and recipes for success.

As you progress, keep in mind the fundamental principles outlined in this cookbook:

1. Balanced Nutrition: Prioritize balanced nutrition by choosing nutrient-dense foods that promote your recovery and overall well-being. Incorporating lean proteins, healthy fats, and fiber-rich vegetables and fruits into your diet is essential.

2. Mindful Eating: Practice mindful eating by listening to your body's hunger and fullness cues. Take your time while eating, fully enjoy each mouthful, and stay focused during meals.

3. Hydration and Activity: Stay adequately hydrated by drinking plenty of water and including regular physical activity in your routine. This will help enhance your metabolism and promote overall well-being.

4. Overcoming Challenges: Successfully address food intolerances, effectively manage emotional eating, and develop healthy coping mechanisms to navigate obstacles and stay on track with your goals.

5. Preparation and Planning: Embrace the power of weekly meal planning, smart grocery shopping, and efficient meal prep techniques to guarantee a constant supply of nutritious meals and snacks.

It's important to remember that everyone's journey is different, so giving yourself time and patience is crucial as you adjust to your new lifestyle. Celebrate your progress, no matter how small, and seek support from friends, family, or support groups when needed.

We trust that this cookbook has provided delicious recipes and valuable insights to make your post-surgery diet pleasurable and long-lasting. We wish you ongoing success, good health, and lasting happiness. Embrace the journey and savor every delightful meal you encounter!

Recipes Index

B

Baked Chicken Parmesan 108

Baked Chicken Thighs 120

Baked Cod with Herbs 102

Baked Eggplant Parmesan 113

Baked Falafel with Tzatziki 123

Baked Salmon with Lemon 98

Baked Tilapia with Herbs 116

Baked Tofu with Soy Sauce 106

Beef and Broccoli Stir-Fry 119

Beef and Vegetable Stew 110

Broccoli Cheddar Soup 15

C

Carrot Turmeric Soup 32

Chicken and Vegetable Stir-Fry 101

Chicken Caesar Salad 115

Chicken Fajita Bowl 111

Clear Chicken Bone Broth 16

Clear Vegetable Broth 28

Coconut Carrot Ginger Soup 35

Coconut Curry Lentil Soup 14

Cottage Cheese with Pineapple 68

Cottage Cheese with Tomato 80

Creamy Asparagus Soup 36

Creamy Carrot Ginger Soup 11

Creamy Cauliflower Mash 44

Creamy Cauliflower Soup 22

Creamy Corn and Poblano Soup 31

Cucumber Dill Soup 37

F

French Onion Soup 39

G

Garlic and Herb Broth 33

Gazpacho 40

Greek Yogurt with Honey 70

Green Pea and Mint Soup 30

Grilled Chicken Breast 97

Grilled Pork Tenderloin 118

Grilled Salmon Salad 122

Grilled Shrimp Skewers 105

Grilled Vegetable Skewers 109

L

Lemon Herb Chicken Soup 18

Lemon Lentil Soup 38

M

Mashed Avocado with Lime 71

Mashed Banana and Avocado 51

Mashed Banana with Yogurt 77

Mashed Pear and Ginger 62

Mashed Pumpkin with Spices 57

Mashed Sweet Potatoes 42

Minted Pea Soup 19

Miso Soup with Tofu 34

Moroccan Chickpea Soup 20

Mushroom Barley Broth 21

P

Pumpkin Apple Soup 29

Pureed Beets with Orange 58

Pureed Black Beans with Cilantro 53

Pureed Carrot and Ginger 43

Pureed Cauliflower and Cheese 59

Pureed Chicken and Vegetable 50

Pureed Eggplant and Garlic 63

Pureed Green Beans with Garlic 45

Pureed Lentil and Spinach 60

Pureed Lentil and Tomato 48

Pureed Peas and Mint 47

Pureed Spinach and Cheese 54

Pureed Squash and Sage 65

Pureed Sweet Potato and Coconut 61

Pureed Tomato and Basil 64

Pureed Turkey with Herbs 52

Pureed Zucchini and Basil 55

Q

Quinoa and Veggie Salad 104

R

Roasted Red Pepper Soup 26

Roasted Turkey Breast 99

S

Silky Butternut Squash Puree 46

Silky Butternut Squash Soup 13

Smooth Apple and Cinnamon 49

Smooth Mango and Yogurt 56

Soft Baked Apple with Cinnamon 74

Soft Baked Fish with Herbs 85

Soft Baked Pear with Nutmeg 83

Soft Baked Potato with Cheese 88

Soft Baked Sweet Potato 78

Soft Black Bean Salad 94

Soft Boiled Eggs 72

Soft Cauliflower Mash 93

Soft Cooked Lentils 81

Soft Cooked Oatmeal 76

Soft Cooked Polenta 91

Soft Cooked Quinoa 86

Soft Mango Smoothie Bowl 90

Soft Poached Salmon 69

Soft Roasted Beet Salad 89

Soft Roasted Squash 79

Soft Scrambled Eggs 67

Soft Spinach Frittata 95

Soft Steamed Broccoli 82

Soft Steamed Carrots 92

Soft Steamed Green Beans 87

Soft Tofu Scramble 84

Soft Tofu with Soy Sauce 75

Spicy Black Bean Soup 25

Stuffed Bell Peppers 100

Stuffed Portobello Mushrooms 112

Stuffed Zucchini Boats 107

Sweet Potato Coconut Soup 24

T

Thai Coconut Lemongrass Soup 23

Tomato Basil Broth 12

Tomato Florentine Soup 27

Tuna Salad with Yogurt 73

Turkey and Avocado Wrap 114

Turkey and Veggie Skillet 124

Turkey Meatballs 103

V

Veggie and Hummus Wrap 117

Veggie and Quinoa Bowl 121

Velvety Spinach and Potato Soup 17